PSYCHOTHERAPY
in CLINICAL PRACTICE

Psychodynamic Theory for Clinicians

PSYCHOTHERAPY
in CLINICAL PRACTICE

Psychodynamic Theory for Clinicians

DAVID BIENENFELD, M.D.
Professor and Vice Chair
Department of Psychiatry
Wright State University
Dayton, Ohio

Acquisitions Editor: Charley Mitchell
Managing Editor: Lisa Kairis
Project Manager: Nicole Walz
Senior Manufacturing Manager: Ben Rivera
Senior Marketing Manager: Adam Glazer
Creative Director: Doug Smock
Cover Designer: Louis Fuiano
Production Services: Schawk, Inc.
Printer: R.R. Donnelley—Crawfordsville

© 2006 by Lippincott Williams & Wilkins
530 Walnut Street
Philadelphia, PA 19106
LWW.com

Library of Congress Cataloging-in-Publication Data

Bienenfeld, David.
    Psychodynamic psychotherapy : psychotherapy in clinical practice / David Bienenfeld.
        p. ; cm.
    Includes bibliographical references and index.
    ISBN 0-7817-9949-X (alk. paper)
    1. Psychodynamic psychotherapy. 2. Psychoanalysis. I. Title.
    [DNLM: 1. Psychoanalytic Theory—Case Reports. 2. Psychoanalytic Therapy—methods—Case Reports.
WM 460 B588p 2006]
RC489.P72B52 2006
616.89′14—dc22
                                                                                    2005016150

10 9 8 7 6 5 4 3 2 1

Contents

To Chana Rochel and Eliezer
My beloved children,
my lights, my inspiration

"The extent to which one is unable to explain a concept indicates the extent to which he does not understand it himself. Let one never fool himself into thinking that he understands a concept and merely has difficulty explaining it."

—Rabbi Chaim Soloveitchik

Don't Skip This Introduction

WHY LEARN PSYCHODYNAMIC THEORY?

Those of us who come to learn about psychotherapy do so because we are stimulated by the practice of the art. The intimacy of connection to suffering human beings requesting our help, the unparalleled satisfaction of facilitating emotional healing by our personal interventions, these are our motivations. By comparison, the study of metapsychology, the examination of terms, hypotheses, and models crafted by those who have come before us, seems quite dry and abstract. It is altogether appropriate that the bulk of literature about psychodynamic therapy focuses on technique, on what we say and do to help people get better.

What then is the role and value of theory to the student of psychodynamic psychotherapy? We can learn by analogy. A surgeon spends most of his or her training learning how and where to cut and tie, and most of his or her career perfecting those skills. But it is senseless to begin learning about incisions and sutures before one has achieved some proficiency in anatomy. The effort devoted to this lackluster task provides the basic science groundwork for the subsequent attainment of clinical skills.

The student of psychopharmacology is excited to learn about the therapeutic effects of various medications, their proper dosing, and their creative combinations. Effective acquisition of such knowledge cannot occur by rote or mimicry. Rather, the trainee must have considerable proficiency in the fields of neurophysiology, microanatomy of the central nervous system, physiology of the renal and hepatic systems, and other clinical sciences. To learn these fields, he or she needs to have mastered basic biochemistry and pharmacology, and so on. One cannot become an expert at psychopharmacology without having first learned organic chemistry.

I have undertaken the assembly of this text with the premise that psychodynamic theory is the basic science underlying psychotherapy. Learning technique becomes more sensible when it is grounded in a theoretical framework of how the human mind works in health, in distress, and in illness. The accomplished therapist learns over time how to balance two opposing needs: 1) to listen with enough theory-based prejudice to make some hypothetical sense of a patient's story, and 2) to listen with a fresh and naïve ear, open to messages that do not match the predictions of theory. This text is aimed at fortifying the capacity for the former; the student is encouraged never to lose the latter.

NOTHING IN THIS BOOK IS TRUE

The molecular weight of tin, the acceleration of an object in Earth's gravity, the number of items that 80% of 22-year-old volunteers can recall from a standard story—these are all objectively verifiable entities. We can see on PET scans the evidence of metabolic functions of the parietal lobes under varying circumstances; we can hold a cadaver's thalamus in our hands. We cannot measure a drive, we will never see an ego, and we cannot grasp a self. The concepts about which we will elaborate in these pages have no consensual reality to them. They are ideas and hypotheses only. So of what use are they?

When I look at the night sky, I can see Orion's belt, and I can follow the stars of Ursa Minor to find Polaris and estimate which direction is north. I can use these constellations to help me locate Venus or Mars at the right time of year. I do not believe that there is a ladle, a bear, or a hunter in the sky. But I know that these fictions help me construct order out of what would otherwise be a senseless accumulation of celestial lights, and they can help me get my bearings. The abstract notions of psychodynamic theory serve the same function. Spontaneous communication from a patient will usually include a number of expressed and implied topics. If I listen completely without preconception, I can never do any more than parrot back the patient's words. In order to make useful interventions, I must be able to generate hypotheses; in order to generate hypotheses, I must have a framework of theory that provides the same sort of map to the patient's mind as the zodiac does for the sky.

Thomas S. Kuhn in *The Structure of Scientific Revolutions* described how the conduct of normal science is to amend hypotheses to explain as much observed data as possible. We will see this process at work as we follow the evolution of psychodynamic theories over time. The explanations that worked for Sigmund Freud in treating patients with hysteria in turn-of-the-20th-century Vienna, did not work quite as well, even for him, as patients with compulsive behaviors and paranoid delusions came to his practice; so he modified his own theories. As psychoanalysis proved its benefit to some patients, more and different patients were drawn to seek this treatment. People with much more profound disturbances of perception, thought, and personality stretched the theories to require their evolution, amendment, and occasional replacement. At its core, theory can only be judged pragmatically: How much sense does it make of the material it attempts to explain?

NOTHING IN THIS BOOK IS ORIGINAL

I hope I have created nothing new here. I do not profess to be a developer of novel psychodynamic theories. The purpose of this volume is to assemble the work of the major thinkers in the field in a way that is comprehensible to the therapist and to offer comparisons where they are enlightening. I offer some historical context in the hopes of dispelling the myth that these theories are simply dreamt up out of nowhere.

I have tried to avoid judgment, endorsement, or criticism of any of the theories. It is an unavoidable reality that those who teach and supervise psychotherapy are invested in their own preferred theoretical constructs. The spirited debates that occur at clinical conferences, the heated exchange of ideas in print, all serve to enliven the encounters among points of view and can promote progress in thinking; but they can also be divisive to a degree that discourages students. The summaries presented here are offered as material for the reader to use and evaluate for credibility and utility.

MS. GRAY, MR. BROWN, AND MS. WHITE

At the beginning of this volume are 3 case summaries. Each of the 3 people described represents an individual one might see in the practice of psychotherapy. Each of their problems can be viewed from different perspectives, leading to different conclusions. In every chapter, several of the cases are used to illustrate the application of some of the theoretical principles being described. It is my intent to make the theoretical more tangible by bringing the ideas to bear on familiar clinical problems. Dr. Klafter's outline for case formulations in Appendix C applies the major psychologies to a real patient in a format that allows the reader to implement the theoretical constructs covered in this book.

IT IS JUST A BEGINNING

This volume is deliberately introductory. It provides no exhaustive descriptions of any dimension of psychodynamic theory. I have chosen not to cite references in the text because it is not the intent of this book to prove anything to a scientifically skeptical reader. Instead, I have included recommended readings at the end of each chapter for the reader who wishes to pursue any of the ideas in more depth.

As the reader advances in clinical experience, he or she will raise ever more subtle and interesting questions. The therapist with an active mind will constantly assimilate and evaluate new corners of his or her guiding theories. It is my hope that this volume will be an introduction to a lifetime of learning.

Acknowledgments

I am grateful to many people who have assisted with the creation of this book. **Dr. Jerald Kay**, my chairman and long-time mentor, has fostered my interest in this topic both by his support and by his example, in an environment that often discourages psychodynamic studies. **Sherron Henry**, my program coordinator, has relieved me of many duties that might have impinged on this effort. **Dr. Andrew Klafter** contributed the appendix on psychodynamic formulation; he is an excellent friend and a trustworthy sounding board. **Lisa Kairis** and **Charley Mitchell** have provided the editorial and publishing expertise, and the personal encouragement, to turn my daydream into the book you now hold.

David Bienenfeld, M.D.
Dayton, Ohio

Introduction to Cases

Presented here are the stories of Ms. Gray, Mr. Brown, and Ms. White. While fictional, they represent typical patients with commonly seen problems. Their circumstances have been selected to highlight the abilities of the different theoretical models to provide explanations from their respective points of view.

They will be cited in sidebars through this text. Each case will be used as an illustration several times from assorted perspectives. The reader may find it useful to apply different models for each instance.

CASES

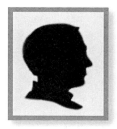

MR. BROWN

Mr. Brown is a 42-year-old married man who has been in weekly psychotherapy for about a year. He came originally because of anxiety, which he related to several sources: His oldest daughter was beginning college, and he was anxious about his ability to support her and his family financially. His wife was angry at him because he had recently withdrawn his name from the competition for a better-paying job in his company, and matters between the couple were tense.

Mr. Brown was the son of a successful businessman, who had high expectations of both himself and those around him. His mother was quiet and passive, and the parents' marriage was unemotional and sometimes strained. Mr. Brown's older brother had been quite successful in school and sports; the patient, somewhat less so. In his recollection, the brother had been clearly favored by the father, while Mr. Brown himself was much closer with his mother.

He had been socially shy in high school and college. While his brother attended an Ivy League university, Mr. Brown attended a state school, where he was an average student despite his above average intelligence. After college, he enrolled in graduate school for business but dropped out several courses short of his master of business administration degree.

He held multiple jobs in business, but his pattern was to rise as a candidate for promotion to management, then to withdraw or sabotage the effort. He recognized this pattern in himself but was unable to explain it. He could identify that something about the process of competition or the prospect of promotion made him nervous and frightened him away from completing the effort.

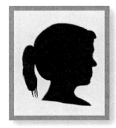

MS. GRAY

Ms. Gray is a 29-year-old woman who came to therapy 4 months ago because she was depressed about her relationship with her boyfriend of the past year, Michael. She describes feeling frustrated and angry. Michael is a binge drinker who is often

1

who is often verbally abusive even when he is not drinking and has been physically abusive occasionally when drunk. She met Michael 2 months after the end of a previous relationship, when she was feeling depressed enough to consider suicide. "I know this relationship is bad for me," she acknowledges, "but I feel as if I'd be too lonely without him, and he can be so nice most of the time."

Ms. Gray was an only child whose father was also alcoholic. She remembers seeing her father beat her mother, who was generally "passive." There are many blanks in her own memory as she has tried to recall her childhood in therapy. She does remember a teacher in fifth grade, Mrs. Hawkins, who felt like a reliable confidante. "I could tell her anything. I really trusted her. When fifth grade was over, I felt like there was a big hole in my life." During adolescence, she used drugs and alcohol sporadically and commonly engaged in risky behavior. She was uneasy about boys, wanting their company, but often ending up feeling abused by them. She married at age 17, but divorced after less than 2 years when her husband left her. At that time, she attempted suicide by overdose of over-the-counter sleeping pills. She finished high school and college and has been gainfully employed at multiple jobs, few lasting more than a year. "Every job I've had, I start with such high expectations, and I'm always disappointed. People just don't keep their promises."

Since the suicide attempt at age 19, she has been receiving antidepressant and anti-anxiety medications, which sometimes help with her sleep and energy but have never addressed her underlying hopelessness, fear, and anger. Until the current therapy, she has never engaged in intensive psychotherapy.

She came to the intake session apprehensive about engaging or trusting the psychiatrist. By the end of the first session, she said, "No one has ever listened to me so closely before. I really think you understand me." Sessions frequently begin with her reports of the turmoil of the preceding week. She often asks for advice. When the psychiatrist refrains from offering advice, she is resentful at his withholding; when he has offered suggestions, she has returned angry that the advice didn't work.

Two weeks ago, the psychiatrist announced his upcoming vacation (his first of this therapy), starting four weeks later. Ms. Gray shrugged off the announcement. The next session, she reported that "things are as bad as they were before I ever came to see you." Her depression and her sense of being trapped in the relationship were intense, and the patient seemed unapproachable with empathic reflections. Any interpretations were met with scorn. Ms. Gray insisted on a change in her medication and demanded lorazepam for her agitation and insomnia. The psychiatrist prescribed 21 tablets of 1mg lorazepam for the subsequent week. At the next session, Ms. Gray was tearful and helpless. Near the end of the session, she said, "This is pointless. I really want to die. I'm going to drive my car into a phone pole on the way home."

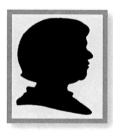

MS. WHITE

Ms. White is a 56-year-old woman who came to therapy on the recommendation of a friend because she was feeling depressed. She describes her depression as "feeling lost." She has little motivation for anything but necessary activities, and she gets less pleasure than she used to from those pursuits in which she does engage. She cannot find much purpose or meaning in her life. She finds herself acting "cranky" with her 62-year-old husband and is less excited than she thinks she should be about their upcoming 35th wedding anniversary. She has never before sought therapy or "nerve medicine" and has never previously thought of herself as especially depressed or anxious.

Ms. White readily identifies two recent developments that preceded her current dysphoria. Last year, her youngest daughter graduated high school and went to college out of town. The Whites have five children, all of them living more than 100 miles away, who keep in frequent and supportive contact by telephone. Ms. White has always taken great pride and satisfaction in her role as a mother. "I know what they mean by the 'empty nest,'" she said at her first session. "The house seems huge and vacant with Suzie gone. I didn't think I'd ever miss doing her laundry, but I do."

The second development was her husband's early retirement this year. He had been a mid-level executive who helped out some but mostly left the household and family duties to his wife. Their marriage has been a happy one, devoid of any but the expectable incidents of conflict and tension. Mr. White would have preferred to work a few years longer but was enticed into retiring early. Ms. White perceives him to be a little bitter. He spends a good deal of time with his friends and community activities but is still at home many more hours per week than he had ever been before. "I know it's his home as much as mine, but it feels like he's always underfoot. Last week he rearranged all the shelves in my laundry room. He tries to save me effort by making his own lunch but leaves an awful mess behind."

Ms. White was the product of a stable family. Her parents were "very traditional"; her father worked in a factory and her mother kept house. She remembers that she could always trust her family to take care of her and recalls admiring both her parents for their stability. Ms. White graduated college and taught elementary school until the birth of her first son then stayed home. She has been a member of her church and several social organizations but was never very committed to any of them.

As a patient, Ms. White is regular and prompt in attending her sessions. She almost never disagrees with her therapist, even when he is uncertain bout the correctness of his interventions. She feels guilty about her current depression. "I shouldn't resent my husband; he's worked so hard for all of us. And I wouldn't want my daughter to know how much I miss her. I wouldn't want her to feel bad about leaving home."

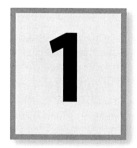

Drive Psychology

"Passions are generally roused from great conflict."

—Titus Livius (Livy)

LEARNING OBJECTIVES

The reader will be able to:

1. Define the fundamental hypotheses of psychodynamic psychology.
2. Describe the major functional units of drive psychology, including:
   a. The drives.
   b. The systems unconscious, preconscious, and conscious.
   c. The structures id, ego, and superego.
3. Outline the Oedipal crisis.

HISTORICAL ORIGINS OF PSYCHOANALYSIS

The roots of psychodynamic thought and practice arguably were established in the office of the neurologist. By the late 19th century, European physicians were intrigued with the mystery of the many "hysterics" who came to see them. These hysterics were usually young women and they described assortments of symptoms including fainting, paralysis, and sensory disturbances.

Because of the centrality of neurological symptoms in their presentations, these patients often consulted neurologists, who were dismayed not only by the inexplicability of the symptoms, but by the often flighty and theatrical style of the sufferers. Clinicians were intrigued by the reported success achieved by Jean Martin Charcot and Hippolyte Bernheim, who were able to relieve hysterical symptoms using the recently disseminated technique of hypnosis. Bernheim, believing that hysteria was a product of suggestion, would implant posthypnotic suggestions that would reverse the symptoms of hysteria, if only temporarily. Among those who flocked to Bernheim's clinic in 1888 was a Viennese neurologist, Sigmund Freud (1856–1939).

Born in a small town in the Austrian crown land of Moravia, Freud was the son of a lively wool merchant and his wife. The family moved to Vienna when Freud was about 5 years old. He was a brilliant student throughout his schooling, and a career in medicine was only natural for him. At the University of Vienna he worked in the laboratory of the renowned physiologist Ernst Brücke. In an era when the science of medicine was still tainted with remnants of folk wisdom and mystical philosophies, Brücke maintained that all forces in an organism could be reduced to the known physical and chemical ones. This notion of reductionism appealed to Freud, and he would spend much of his career trying to reduce psychological phenomena to their neurological bases, although he ultimately gave up that effort.

Freud's particular interest was in neurophysiologic research, but opportunities in that field were scarce, so he entered the practice of clinical neurology. Brücke arranged for Freud to study both with Charcot in Paris and with Bernheim in Nancy. Returning to Vienna, he assisted Dr. Josef Breuer. One of Breuer's patients displayed numerous symptoms of a hysterical nature, which emerged first when she was taking care of her dying father. Notably, she would also experience states she called "clouds," which Breuer labeled as "spontaneous hypnosis." In these states, she could relate her fantasies and often felt transiently better. When her recollections related her feelings to the meaning of a symptom, the relief was more sustained. Breuer and Freud hypothesized that every hysterical symptom has its origin in some psychologically traumatic event, and when the meaning of the symptoms is revealed, the patient loses the need to experience them.

This patient was identified as "Anna O." when her case was featured in *Studies in Hysteria* by Freud and Breuer in 1895. She was overly fond of Breuer and developed a symptom of hysterical pregnancy, believing Breuer to be the father of her child. Breuer, a married man, abruptly ended her treatment and turned her care over to Freud. Freud took her further in her "chimney sweeping," as she called the talking cure, and he discovered a wealth of sexual motivations underlying the hysterical processes.

As a footnote, Anna O., whose real name was Bertha Pappenheim, completed her treatment and became the first social worker in Germany and a vocal proponent of women's suffrage. Freud subsequently took Bernheim's technique a step further, discovering that if he allowed his patients to recall the events surrounding the origins of their hysterical symptoms under hypnosis, the symptoms would remit for much longer than with suggestion only, and sometimes permanently. Before long, Freud abandoned hypnosis altogether and encouraged patients simply to remember without censorship. Thus psychoanalysis was born.

THE FUNDAMENTAL HYPOTHESES OF PSYCHOANALYSIS

Implicit in the cure of hysterics using recollection of forgotten experiences were two notions that formed the *fundamental hypotheses* of psychoanalysis:

1. Mental activity is not random, but each process in the mind is linked to thoughts and events that preceded it (*psychic determinism*).
2. The greater part of mental activity proceeds outside conscious awareness (in the *dynamic unconscious*).

The ability to assign meaning to the seemingly random symptoms of hysterics made psychic determinism an attractive hypothesis, since an object of science is to explain what seems inexplicable. The clinical cures (even if transient) that resulted from the communication of these meanings to the sufferers further bolstered the credibility of this notion. With enough mental effort and creativity, it is possible to assign meaning to all of our thoughts, feelings, behaviors, dreams, and mistakes.

To do so, however, often requires stretching the thread of motivation through territory that is inconsistent with conscious thought and recollection. The principle of psychic determinism thus necessitates the existence of a dynamic unconscious. If all our mental activity is linked to other mental processes, but we cannot see most of these links, then there must be a world of mental activity unavailable to the conscious mind. Although many of the specifics of Sigmund Freud's derivations have been modified or challenged, these two fundamental principles remain at the bedrock of all psychodynamic theories. While Schopenhauer, Nietzsche, Goethe, Schiller, and others in the arts and sciences had acknowledged the existence of mental life beyond awareness, it was Freud who first gave it substantive recognition and described it in scientific detail. And since psychology at the end of the 19th century had already described much about memory, intellect, and other functions of the conscious mind, it would be in the realm of the unconscious that Freud and his followers would have the greatest contributions to make.

THE DRIVES AND LEVELS OF CONSCIOUS AWARENESS

Freud first described three systems of awareness: conscious (system Cs), preconscious (system PCs), and unconscious (system UCs) reflecting, respectively, decreasing levels of immediate awareness. (See Table 1-1.)

These systems contain tempests of mental activity, so what is the source of energy for all this thinking and feeling? In Freud's formulation, the energy springs from the *drives*. The drives are comparable to instincts in animals—biologically determined forces that promote the promulgation of the individual and the species. The term *instinct*, however, includes the behavior and motor activity resulting from the biological urge. In humans, the drives are only the sense of compulsion or urge toward some goal; the activity is separate. In his first formulation, Freud, consistent with the Darwinian paradigm of the times, postulated a *sexual* (reproductive) drive and a self-preservative drive. He soon dropped the latter and for the greater part of three decades elaborated his theories around a single sexual drive. This drive propels the human organism toward reproduction, connection,

TABLE 1-1	*Systems of Awareness*	
System	**Definition**	**Example**
Conscious (Cs)	Mental activity completely within immediate awareness	Greeting a friend by name
Preconscious (PCs)	Mental activity available to conscious awareness, but not in conscious attention at this moment	Knowing a friend's name without having to recall it right now
Unconscious (UCs)	Mental activity concealed beyond conscious awareness, making itself known by indirect manifestations	- Calling a friend by the wrong name because of some perceived but forgotten insult - Dreaming about a distorted representative of the friend

and afffection. By 1922, Freud was unable to explain the wealth of conflict and turmoil he observed in mental life on the basis of a single drive and postulated a second, the *aggressive drive.* This drive promotes destruction and disconnection.

The drives themselves are beyond conscious awareness, even though their names reflect conscious urges. They are biologically propelled urges. The aggression a person feels toward someone he or she hates, and the attraction he or she feels toward a love object, are drive manifestations or *drive derivatives,* but they are not the drives themselves.

In animals, instinct directs activity and every instinctual urge is either satisfied or given up. In people, the drives are purely mental entities. The pressure of a drive creates in the person a sense of excitation or tension. It is the natural state of the human animal to minimize this tension, and we do so either by direct gratification or by some other mode of accommodation. (We will see later in this chapter how these accommodations are managed.) Further, every thought, emotion, or fantasy embodies a mix of both sexual and aggressive drives. No love is without hostility or fear; no anger is without affection or envy. With just these simple principles in place, the mind is now a very active site: Sexual and aggressive

gressive drives coexist, often uncomfortably; if the drive impulse cannot be directly satisfied, the person is suspended in a state of tension and unfulfilled excitement; and this whole commotion is occurring outside the narrow bounds of conscious awareness.

MS. GRAY experienced an early childhood of intense emotions connected to both *sexual and aggressive drives*. Connected naturally to both parents by innate urges for closeness, she was buffeted by her father's violence and probably resented her mother's passivity. Especially at such an early age, the emotions connected to experience were too intense for her to accommodate, so she could not establish lasting memory traces. Her memories instead were relegated to her *unconscious*, accounting for her inability to recollect much of her early life.

THE STRUCTURAL MODEL

The systems UCs, PCs, and Cs are the elements of the *topographic model* of the mind. By itself, the topographic description cannot portray how the drives operate and what directs movement among the topographic systems. It thus falls short of explanatory power to account for many of the ideas and symptoms of Freud's analysands. This explanation is elucidated in Freud's later *structural model*. The structures he defined are id, ego, and superego:

- *Id* is the most primitive mental structure. It contains sexual and aggressive drive derivatives in their most unalloyed form. Because it originates in the earliest stage of mental development, it is nonverbal; even more importantly, id precedes the acquisition of memory so it has no sense of time and cannot construct a chronological narrative or a sense of continuity of self or other.
- *Ego* is the structure that achieves gratification for the drives—directly when possible, diverted or delayed when necessary. Ego's first capacities are those of control over motor function, such as putting the finger into the mouth, or later, walking and talking. Ego's cognitive capabilities allow for the existence of memory, which then makes delayed gratification of id impulses possible.

- *Superego* is the structure that regulates acceptable ways for drives to be satisfied or discharged. It consists of both ideals toward which ego strives and conscience, which limits drive-motivated behavior. At first, the child blindly internalizes the values of parents and other close figures. True consolidation of the superego, however, only occurs as the result of the Oedipal situation (which we will examine below).

PSYCHOLOGICAL DEVELOPMENT

The mind of the newborn infant consists entirely of id. The child experiences pleasant and unpleasant physical sensations such as hunger and satiety, cold and warmth. He or she is driven toward gratification of id impulses, the earliest of which center on nursing and feeding. But the infant is completely at the mercy of his or her environment and can do nothing personally to gratify the urges. With maturation of the nervous system comes the ability to distinguish self from other, and the ability to manipulate parts of the self. So the child realizes that he or she can put his or her thumb into his or her mouth and at least partly gratify the urge to suck. Almost simultaneous is the pleasant sensation that the thumb has of being sucked, so the infant has become both the agent and the recipient of id gratification; this passage is the beginning of the ego. (In Freud's words, "The ego is first a body ego.")

Before long, the child acquires the ability to communicate, and the developing consciousness harbors the awareness that crying often produces relief. This ability will mature into the capacity for speech, just as motor skills develop to include the achievements of crawling and walking. Ego directs these abilities toward satisfaction of drive urges and minimization of discomfort.

Similarly, the growing brain acquires the capacity for memory. While the newborn is only aware of his or her mother when she is immediately in the child's presence, the nine-month-old can remember that mother exists even when she is not there. Memory is the foundation for ego's capacity for fantasy: When mother is not there, baby can imagine her presence and soothe himself or herself until mother really does arrive. In structural terms, this function is known as *delayed gratification,* an ego milestone. Ego is now able to serve id with mental tools in addition to motor skills.

Freud defined two types of mental function to describe the activities of the growing mind. Each refers both to a set of cognitive patterns, and to the ways in which drive energy is allocated and discharged:

- *Primary process* is the earliest, inborn style of mental activity. It seeks immediate gratification of drive urges, and it is extremely fluid in its cognitive associations.
- *Secondary process* is characteristic of the mature ego. It has the ability to delay drive discharge, and its cognitive rules are more rigid. (See Table 1-2.)

TABLE 1-2 | *Cognitive Features of Primary Process*

Feature	*Definition*	*Example from Dream or "Slip"*
Absence of negatives	All statements and emotions are framed in the affirmative, without conditions or qualifications. Only context determines true meaning.	A man says, "I want you to go shopping with your friends" when he wants her to stay home, and intended to say, "I don't want you to go. . . "
Equality of opposites	Images and ideas of antithetical difference appear together, and may substitute one for another	Despised gym teacher represents beloved art teacher in a memory
Representation by analogy or allusion	Parts of an object or memory stand for the whole. Similar images are freely exchanged for each other.	An image of a swing set represents time spent playing with father in childhood
Fluidity of form	Images or sensory impressions may be used to represent words or ideas	Sensation of shivering in the cold represents anger at the blind date who left a man standing in the snow and waiting
Absence of time	There is no logical or historical sequence. Past, present, and even future are as one.	Current husband shows up in dream of early family life

All along, the objects of the drives change and grow in a pattern that Freud assumed to be biologically determined:

- The *oral phase* of drive development occupies most of the first year of life. The infant is focused on oral gratification of sexual drives (not yet separated from the pleasure of feeding) through sucking and of aggressive drives through biting.
- The second and third years of life constitute the *anal phase* of development. The child gets sexual pleasure out of both the retention and elimination of feces, and aggressive gratification out of withholding and depositing feces. This phase is important for its contribution to the child's sense of mastery of his or her body and the ability to control the environment.
- The *phallic phase* usually begins in the third or fourth year of life. Now the child experiences genital sources of pleasure and recognizes the differences between boys and girls. Masturbation is a significant source of sexual gratification and urination can be an aggressive outlet. This is the last phase of early childhood psychosexual development, and blends into the developmental tasks of latency, adolescence, and adulthood.

Like all the developmental schemes we will examine, Freud's does not proceed in rigid lockstep. Failures in the environment or traumatic situations can cause manifestations of one phase to persist into the next, a phenomenon called *fixation*. Fixation affects how character traits are displayed through subsequent development and adult life. Anxiety-provoking circumstances can prompt temporary *regression* to an earlier phase. And neither oral nor anal appetites ever disappear completely; they persist in distorted forms even in healthy individuals.

Character Styles

Whether due to fixation in the face of frustration, or to regression in the face of anxiety, each of these phases can shape adult personality. Clearly, influences of fixation tend to be more persistent than those of regression.

- The *oral passive* personality is a result of frustrated needs to suckle in early infancy. These people tend to be overly dependent on others and seek "oral gratification" through eating, drinking, and smoking.

■ The *oral aggressive* personality stems from frustrated attempts at teething, for example when the mother rejects the baby for biting her nipple and attempts to wean him or her too early. In adulthood, such people are verbally aggressive, sarcastic, and argumentative.

■ The *anal expulsive* (or *anal aggressive*) personality is the product of a childhood in which the parents are overly subservient to the toddler's toilet training, giving rewards for desired behavior and suffering transparently when the child fails. Adults with this character style are sloppy and disorganized. They may be overly generous or cruel and destructive.

■ The *anal retentive* personality is the product of overly strict toilet training. The parents use punishment or shame, and the child responds (or retaliates) by holding in feces at all costs. Such children likely grow up to be stingy, compulsively neat, stubborn, and rigid.

■ The *phallic personalities* are more complicated and less well-defined. They originate in the Oedipal phase described below. If the boy is rejected by his mother and threatened by his father, he may maintain a sense of inadequacy and either withdraw from heterosexual dealings, or he may overreact and become the macho man (the so-called "Don Juan complex"). A girl rejected by father and intimidated by mother will similarly either withdraw or become overly feminine.

On the other hand, if the boy is favored by mother over a weak father, or if the daughter is favored by father over his wife, there is no need to compete. The boy may grow to be self-impressed and/or effeminate; the girl, vain and/or masculine.

THE OEDIPAL CRISIS

The period from ages 4 through 6 is the most tempestuous passage in the Freudian scheme. The body has developed phallic urges. The ego can avail itself of an intellect that perceives, understands, and remembers a great deal, and which can ambulate and communicate. Unrestrained, the ego would devour pleasures for the gratification of id. At the same time, the youngster has incorporated a primitive sense of right and wrong, of reward and punishment, and of societal norms. The stage is now set for the passionate drama of the *Oedipal crisis.*

Oedipus was the tragic hero of Greek mythology whose inescapable fate was to murder the man he did not know to be his father and to marry the woman he did not know to be his mother. Upon discovering the truth, he was driven by guilt and shame to blind himself. In this tale, Freud read a universal pattern of development.

Every child, with the inexorable maturation of phallic urges, comes to experience strong sexual attraction to the mother. (We will deal first with what happens to boys during this period.) The 4-year-old boy, excited by his mother, wants to achieve physical intimacy with her. Ego, however, recognizes some difficulties in gratifying this id drive. First, there is the presence of the father, who is noticeably more powerful and unlikely to relinquish possession of his wife. Second, (Freud presumed) the boy has noticed that girls and women lack the penis that he and father have. His fantasy is that they have lost their penises and that he will lose his, too, if father discovers his rivalry for mother. The boy's envy and hate for father and his wish to have father out of the way, is the equivalent (in fantasy) of murder. With this wish, the fear of castration grows even more intense.

Ego has already achieved the ability to grow by virtue of *identification,* of becoming like a figure in the environment. To cope with the potentially overwhelming anxiety of the Oedipal conflict, ego identifies with father, a mechanism known as *identification with the aggressor.* By assimilating father's strength, the boy retains some sense of self confidence. Further, by owning the restrictions of parental morality, the boy is relieved of some of the fear of revenge from outside. This assimilation of goals and conscience is the beginning of the final element of structural theory, the *superego.* Superego contains modified and displaced urges from id, transforming them into socially acceptable ideals and providing alternative routes of gratification. Ego gains by having id energy thus diverted, but faces a different challenge because it must now juggle the drives of id on the one hand and the restrictions of shame, doubt, guilt, and punishment from superego on the other. All the ingredients are now present for the emergence of psychic conflict and neurotic psychopathology, as we will examine later.

MR. BROWN retains his wish for *Oedipal* union with his mother, which would require displacing the father. In the adult world, job accomplishment is the symbolic equivalent of identification with the father and brings the promise of Oedipal union with mother. Each approach to external success, however, is perceived by his *superego* as an emergence of *aggressive* urges toward his rival. Superego reacts by mobilizing self-doubt and fear of retribution.

Freud's theories of girls' psychosexual development were never fully satisfying to him and have only lost credibility with the passage of time. The little girl's transit through the Oedipal maze is described here for completeness: The girl, too, is sexually attracted to her mother. However, she notices that she does not even have the penis that father has and concludes that she has lost it, or never had it. She is enraged at mother for allowing her to be so deprived, and copes with this rage by identifying with mother and secondarily developing an attraction to father. Seeing that father will not allow himself to be stolen from mother, she is forced to suppress or redirect her id drives. The development of her superego is driven not by castration anxiety but by penis envy. The methodological, clinical, and political shortcomings of this model are obvious and will not be further elaborated.

SYNTHESIS OF SYSTEMS AND STRUCTURES

By this point, the model has three dimensions:

1. Drives are aggressive or sexual and provide the energy
2. Thoughts and feelings are contained in the systems unconscious, preconscious, and conscious
3. The apparatus that puts these drives to work consists of id, ego, and superego

These elements are sufficient to describe a rich texture of mental activity. It is important to remember that the structural model does not displace the topographic model, rather it supplements it. Elements of id, ego, and superego operate in conscious, preconscious, and unconscious forms, although ego of course dominates conscious life.

The balancing act that ego performs between the drives of id and the demands of superego and reality forces the develop-

ment of an array of *defense mechanisms* that would be elaborated
by Freud's successors (Chapter 3). During sleep, when the demands of reality and society are absent, when the energy of the
defenses is lowered, the demands of id and the reactions of superego are symbolized in the elaborate life of dreams. The constant juggling of drives and defenses is never perfect, and bits of
disguised id urge break out as *parapraxes,* the errors we have
come to know as "Freudian slips." And, almost inevitably, the
conflict inherent in the system leads to psychopathology, as
elaborated in Chapter 7.

DREAMS

Sigmund Freud described dreams as "the royal road to the unconscious." *The Interpretation of Dreams* (1900) was perhaps his most
revolutionary contribution. Popular images of classical psychoanalysis almost invariably include references to dream interpretation, and indeed the study of dreams retains a central position
in drive psychology. Popular culture of the early 20th century was
likely to regard dreams as portents of the future. Psychology had
yet to develop a coherent explanation for dreams. Although
Freud's formulations have been subject to considerable criticism,
and to substantial revision even within the field of drive psychology, his efforts were groundbreaking, and the essentials persist in
the practice of drive-based psychoanalysis into the present.

   Although most dreams remembered by adults are so confusing that they tend to be disturbing, drive psychology maintains
that their purpose is to protect sleep. The dream protects the
sleeper from interruptions stemming from bodily discomfort such
as pain, cold, or hunger; from conscious preoccupations left over
from the day's thinking; and from unconscious urges originating
in the id. A review of some of the relevant terms will facilitate our
understanding of this process.

   The events and images experienced by the dreamer are the
manifest dream content. (They may or may not be remembered after waking, but are considered to be conscious during sleep.) The
thoughts and sensations that threaten to wake the dreamer are
the *latent dream content.* The unconscious mental operations that
keep the latent content out of awareness and fashion the images
of the manifest content are called *dream work* (Figure 1-1).

The latent dream content has several components:

1. Nocturnal sensory stimuli, such as bodily sensations noted above, as well as noises, winds, and other intrusions
2. The preoccupations of waking life, including the worries and fears that one would rather be rid of, often called *day residue*
3. Repressed id impulses, both libidinal and aggressive, pressing for fulfillment

It is this latter group, the repressed id impulses, which is the vital and essential part of the latent dream content, the source of most of its psychic energy. In fact, bodily sensations or daytime preoccupations alone are not sufficient to wake the sleeper or even to produce dreams by themselves. They must enlist some element of the repressed id in order to create a dream.

Freud relied on early childhood dreams to formulate his model of dreams in adulthood. (One may argue with his methodology, since he never analyzed young children himself; but our purpose here is only to delineate his conclusions.) The manifest content of dreams of early childhood, he concluded, all represented straightforward fulfillment of id wishes. It is possible for young children to dream this way because the ego is not yet sufficiently developed to mandate repression of most wishes, and there is no superego to contribute its own levels of anxiety and guilt. So the young child's id achieves partial gratification of its wishes in the manifest dream and loses its power to wake the child. The child may dream of suckling at the breast, so the libidinal energy is contained enough to protect sleep.

Later in childhood, dreams begin to resemble those of adults. They become more divorced from reality and at times are more emotionally disturbing. Here, said Freud, the fantasy of wish fulfillment is still at the core, but the manifest content represents a distortion mandated by other forces. This distortion is the result of dream work. Dream work has two major components:

Latent content is translated into the language of primary process. As described above, primary process has no respect for chronology and allows for liberal symbolic substitution. The medium of dreams is primarily visual; so the primary process seeks an image that is close to the wish-fulfillment fantasy, and usually retains elements of day residue. Because visual images are singular, the dream's representations require *condensation*, a primary process operation involving the combination of several ideas and urges into a single vehicle. Because the primary process is seeking only to give vent to id wishes without disturbing sleep, there is no need for these images to be comprehensible to the conscious mind, and no need for the plot of the dream to make sense to the secondary process.

The ego exerts its defensive force to contain further the representations of id wishes. Since Freud was decades away from formulating the structural model when he published *The Interpretation of Dreams*, he originally employed the term "dream censor," until he later described the ego more fully. The ego is opposed to the emergence of many id wishes into consciousness when the person is awake and must resist these urges in sleep as well. Ego, therefore, makes a "deliberate" effort to disguise the wishes behind unrecognizable images. Further, ego is responsible for mastering those elements of day residue that create guilt, anxiety, or other forms of displeasure. Just as it mounts defense mechanisms during the day, ego mobilizes distortion at night to prevent these unpleasant emotions from intruding on sleep. While the distortions of primary process make dream images unrecognizable in a passive way (i.e., primary process doesn't need the images to be comprehensible), ego defenses do so actively (i.e., the defenses are only successful if the images are undecipherable).

Emotions, too, are subject to such amendment. They are often attenuated, modified, or even replaced by their opposites. Anger may become love, fear may become confidence. Ultimately, the manifest dream is a "compromise formation," in Freud's words, between the opposing forces of the latent content and the defensive operations of the ego.

Contrary to popular myth, drive psychology does not maintain that there is a dictionary of dream images. Trains and snakes are not always penises, mountains and clouds are not always breasts. Even primary process is shaped by experience, and ego certainly is. The specific symbols that wind up in the dream represent particular meanings to the individual dreamer. Dream analysis requires the elucidation of those specific meanings in order to identify the id wishes forcing the dream and the ego mechanisms shaping its content.

MS. WHITE reported that she had been shopping at the mall the previous day attempting to distract herself and had a dream last night that took place in the mall. "I was standing in the atrium, staring with pleasure at the colorful mobile hanging from the skylight. A man, a stranger, walked over from the automatic teller machine and stood next to me. He got progressively closer until he was pressing on me. I turned and hugged him."

Prompted by the therapist for her associations to various elements of the dream, she related that the mobile made her think of a similar one that hung over the crib of her youngest child. The ATM reminded her of the bank where her husband used to work. The therapist hypothesized that Ms. White wished for a return of the days when her children were in their cribs and she could be happy as a mother. The man represented her husband, who left the bank and intruded on her space. Her aggressive urges, unacceptable to her ego, were transformed into an act of apparent affection.

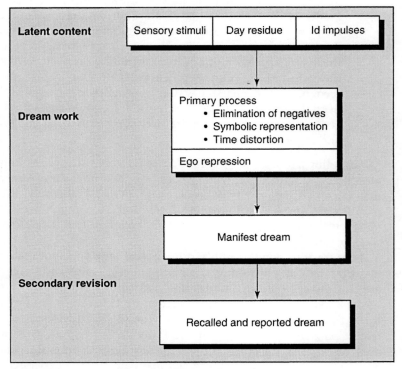

FIGURE 1-1 Freud's Model of Dream Formation.

Even subsequent to waking, the distortion process is not yet complete. Secondary process, now aroused, does not tolerate the garbled, confusing, and incoherent content of the manifest dream, and undertakes immediately to package it more tastefully. The waking ego, both consciously and unconsciously, edits and revises the dream. It makes symbols more recognizable and less idiosyncratic. It inserts order into the dream's chaos and constructs logic to shape the dream's meandering plot. The results of this *secondary revision* only serve to make the real wishes and compromises even less comprehensible behind the façade of rationality.

MISTAKES AND JOKES

Probably every contemporary reader is familiar with the phrase, "Freudian slip." Such mistakes, along with wit and humor, Freud regarded as the "psychopathology of everyday life." These phenomena were further evidence for him that the model he had derived from the analysis of neurotic people was equally valid as a general psychology.

For those revealing mistakes we call "slips," he used the term *Fehlleistungen,* generally translated as *parapraxes,* and the term applies most commonly to errors of the tongue or pen that carry implied psychological significance. In fact, the simplest parapraxis is forgetting. If a person forgets a spouse's birthday or an appointment with the gastroenterologist, he or she may say, "I had no reason to forget," because the reason is unconscious. Such forgetting is a direct manifestation of repression. In order to prevent experiencing the guilt about withholding affection from the spouse or the fear of a colonoscopy, a person may simply forget the related event. In psychoeconomic terms, the energy of the ego is directed against the superego or the id.

Slips of the tongue or pen, the more common and interesting parapraxes, are similar, but they represent a failure of the ego to repress completely the source of anxiety or guilt. The result is that the person expresses in mildly disguised form what he or she unconsciously meant to say. The teacher who calls his or her student a "patient" may be revealing feelings about the student's attitude and behavior.

While the hidden intent may seem to be evident in the content of the slip, such a correlation is only speculative until confirmed or modified by associations and analysis. The form of a slip is frequently determined by primary process. Thus one may find himself or herself unexpectedly uttering a neologism that is the unconscious mind's attempt to disguise anxiety by a process like condensation to fuse words. Primary process connections between images (displacement, representation of the whole by a part, etc.) may shape the mistaken terms or names one uses. Metaphors and poetry use the same mechanisms, with the important difference that they are deliberately chosen, not dictated by the unconscious.

Accidents are another case of parapraxes. By definition they entail no conscious intent, but all actions enabling the accident represent the unconscious at work. In most accidents, the punitive superego creates circumstances of loss or injury out of a need for punishment or restitution.

Humor, particularly wit, involves similar dynamics. It makes use of primary process forms like condensation (necessary for puns) and representation by analogy. To Freud's ear, most wit centers on either hostile or sexual content, reflective of drive urges. Regardless of how clever, a joke is only effective if it has a point. The jokester regresses temporarily to make use of the primary process associations to create the joke. When uttered, it permits a form of gratification of the underlying urge. The listener, too, regresses in order to be able to understand the primary process message, and the urge is gratified for him or her as well. The energy which was used to contain the anxiety is suddenly released as laughter.

NARCISSISM AND OBJECT RELATIONS

The 21st century reader, familiar with a setting in which people seeking psychotherapy usually relate their distress to difficulties with other people, will note that Sigmund Freud's psychology emphasizes individual development and function, attributing only generic roles to parents and others. Since Freud was exploring and explaining the power of the unconscious, it is understandable that he would direct his focus toward the individual. But he was forced to venture into some speculation about how individuals relate to others, if for no other reason than to explain the role of others in individual development. His efforts serve as the beginnings of a theoretical theme that would be much more fully developed by others and as outlined in Chapters 3 through 6.

Anna O.'s much distorted perception of Breuer, a phenomenon that would subsequently acquire the name of *transference*, made it clear even in the earliest phases of psychoanalytic formulation that people perceive others in ways that do not accurately reflect objective reality. Many of the stories Freud heard made him curious about the relationship between reality and perception of others. Freud designated psychologically significant individuals, things and ideas outside the self as *objects*, a term which has become permanent in the psychodynamic vocabulary.

In most of Freud's writing, an object is simply anything to which a drive attaches. It is the nature of the drive that determines the psychological perception of the object. In earliest life, the sexual or libidinal drive is much more powerful and significant than the aggressive drive. Furthermore, at its most primitive, even the sexual drive is not yet coherent; the oral, anal, and phallic characteristics outlined earlier are almost like separate drives. The infant accumulates sets of satisfying and frustrating experiences and even before ego is capable of conscious memory, forms internal images of satisfaction. The images are associated with the conditions under which they formed, including the responsible object. Since the sexual drive is still heterogeneous, the images are similarly fragmented. Such images are termed *part objects;* most classically, the breast that satisfies the oral craving is perceived as an object unto itself, not yet part of the mother to whom it is attached.

At the very earliest, the drives are objectless, since the infant's mind cannot even create an object. As the first direction of libido is autoerotic, the child often gains satisfaction by sucking his or her thumb; and the thumb itself, not yet recognizable as part of the self, becomes an early part object. The breast is the first object outside the self.

As the growing brain amasses experiences, it yields the capacity for memory and, with it, the development of ego as described earlier. Now object relations can assume a different form. The ego, which synthesizes perception, becomes the storehouse for object images. Since the ego's first concern is the self, and since libido's first objects are parts of the self, one of the most important objects the ego can contain is the image of the self. The investment of libido in the image of the self is called *narcissism*, a term which would undergo many modifications in the decades after Freud first presented it. Ego at this point has a new and important power: It can harness libidinal energy and invest it in an internal object image. Freud maintained that, throughout one's life, the majority of libido is narcissistic, and that this narcissism, under most circumstances, is healthy fuel for normal psychological function.

Investment of libidinal energy solely in a narcissistic direction, however, is a losing proposition. Even the infant needs others. Accumulation of experiences with others allows the ego to establish images of objects besides the self. The investment of drive energy in these images is the beginning of object relations. Even years after defining the structural model, Freud put it this way: "Repeated episodes of satisfaction have created an object out of the mother."

Drive energy, however, is a finite sum. Whatever is cathected to one object must be withdrawn from elsewhere. Ego now has an even more powerful capacity, the ability to allocate drive energy, both libidinal and aggressive to object images inside itself. Implicitly, by assigning the drives to the objects, ego can now change the nature of the drives. Also implicit in this zero-sum schema, however, libido invested in objects outside the self must be withdrawn from narcissistic libido.

Psychological health requires relationships with others as whole objects, not part objects. Getting to that stage requires ego to give up self-investment and to integrate the part objects into whole ones. For the infant, the smiling face is a different object from the angry one. Memory must be harnessed for the child to associate the two. The capacity for ambivalence, which begins to accrue from ages 2 to 5, is critical for the assimilation of disparate facets into unified objects. Success or failure in this task determines ultimate happiness in the world of real people.

Learning points

- The drive model of psychology began with Sigmund Freud's studies of hysteria. It emphasizes the primacy of unconscious mental processes in shaping thought and behavior. The energy for mental activity springs from the innate sexual and aggressive drives.
- The topographic model describes the layers of awareness: conscious, preconscious, and unconscious.
- The structural model describes the systems of the mind. Id is the repository of unmodified drive urges; ego is the vehicle by which those urges are gratified, modified, or postponed; and superego is the collection of goals and conscience that shapes the limits of thought and behavior.
- The mechanisms by which ego gratifies or diverts id urges are the defenses.
- Biological maturation dictates a succession of objects to the drives from oral to anal to phallic.
- The Oedipal crisis is the major transition for the developing child, during which the structures and systems are solidified.
- Dreams represent id wishes, distorted by primary process and ego defenses, to provide a unique window into the unconscious mind.

RECOMMENDED READINGS

Brenner C. *An Elementary Textbook of Psychoanalysis* (revised ed.). New York: Anchor Books, 1973.

Dilts SL. *Models of the Mind; A Framework for Biopsychosocial Psychiatry.* Philadelphia: Brunner-Routledge, 2001.

Jacobs M. *Sigmund Freud.* London: Sage Publications, 1992.

Kline P. *Psychology and Freudian Theory: An Introduction.* London: Methuen & Co., 1984.

Meissner WW. *Freud and Psychoanalysis.* South Bend, IN: Notre Dame Press, 2000.

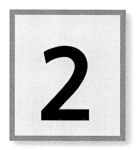

Dissent: Alfred Adler and Carl Jung

"There are two kinds of truths: small truth and great truth. You can recognize a small truth because its opposite is a falsehood. The opposite of a great truth is another great truth."

—*Niels Bohr*

LEARNING OBJECTIVES

The reader will be able to:

1. Define the roles of fictions, superiority, and inferiority in Alfred Adler's theory of development and personality.
2. Describe the importance of social interest, lifestyle, and birth order in Adler's model.
3. Define the collective unconscious and its archetypes in Carl Jung's psychology.
4. Outline Jung's personality typologies.

ROOTS OF DIVISION

By the first decade of the 20th century, Sigmund Freud had achieved a small but intense following that included physicians, clerics, and other intellectuals fascinated by his novel approach to the human condition. The group eventually organized as the Viennese Psycho-Analytic Society. By all accounts, its meetings were quite lively. Today, we can read the evolution of Freud's thinking by following his papers chronologically. He would present these ideas as he was forming them, which promoted spirited discussion at the time. Although Freud fostered such debate, he ran his society in quite a paternalistic fashion. Dissent was tolerated only within narrow limits; those who persisted in disagreement would find themselves subject to disapproval, overt criticism, and even rejection from the group.

Because psychoanalysis still occupied a position at the fringe of medicine, and even psychology, the Society as a whole struggled to achieve public acceptance. Those who were cast out had little hope of winning any influence in medical or intellectual spheres. Of those dissenters, two, Alfred Adler and Carl Jung, achieved renown and their ideas persist even today. (Because their ideas failed to exert profound influence on subsequent development of mainstream psychodynamic thought, this chapter will present their theories on normal function, psychopathology, and therapy rather than postponing the latter two considerations for subsequent chapters.)

Alfred Adler

Alfred Adler (1870–1937) was the third child in his family. He developed rickets early in life and did not begin to walk until age 4. When he was 5 years old, he suffered a near fatal bout of pneumonia; it was upon recovery from this illness that he set his mind on a career as a physician. As a boy, he was an affable, outdoorsy type, known for his energetic competition with his older brother (named Sigmund!). After obtaining his medical degree from the University of Vienna, he began practice as an ophthalmologist and then took up general medical practice. His office was in a part of Vienna across from an amusement park/circus, and many of his patients were circus and sideshow performers who displayed unusual combinations of strengths and deficits.

Adler's interest in psychiatry evolved, and he was attracted to Sigmund Freud's ideas and was invited to join Freud's discussion group in 1907. Because of his social and intellectual skills, Adler was named the first president of the Viennese Psycho-Analytic Society and editor of its newsletter. Despite his closeness to Freud, he took issue with some crucial ideas. Particularly, he saw the sexual drive as more metaphoric than literal and did not see it (in the days before Freud postulated the dual-drive theory) as the only motivator of human behavior. The dispute grew beyond the possibility of resolution, and in 1911, Adler and nine other members resigned to form their own organization.

During World War I, Adler served in the Austrian army and witnessed the ravages of war. His experiences in that conflict gave rise in large part to his emphasis on "social interest" (see below). Much of his postwar work was focused less on treatment of individual psychopathology and more on socially focused interventions, such as training teachers in the psychology of children.

MOTIVATION

Adler, like Freud, sought a single motivating force behind human behavior, but he rejected his mentor's attempts to reduce that motivation to the physiologic level of a "drive." Adler was more attentive to the entirety of personality and sought a more comprehensive model that encompassed social and cultural dimensions as well. He called his model "individual psychology," in the sense that individual means indivisible; i.e., what we would now call a holistic approach.

He began in the Viennese Psycho-Analytic Society by postulating the existence of the "aggression drive." Here, aggression is not precisely the same as what Freud would describe in his later dual-drive theory, but refers to the reaction one has when primary needs such as food, sex, or affection, are frustrated. What Adler described is an inborn tendency to compensatory assertiveness. Freud's fear was that attention to this drive would detract from the centrality of the sexual drive; and the division over this subject led Adler to leave the Society, even though his ideas are consistent with some of Freud's later writings on the drives and instincts.

Aggression drive was too negative in its destructive implications, and Adler began instead to describe "compensation," or the "striving to overcome." Since all individuals have some shortcomings, they naturally attempt to overcome them. Adler believed a great deal of personality could be described by individuals' attempts to compensate for their natural deficiencies. But he became dissatisfied with this model because it suggests that people are primarily the product of their reactions to their problems. His next step was consistent with Friedrich Neitzsche's "will to power," and Adler postulated the "striving for superiority" as an engine of human thought and action. Superiority was a more suitable complex notion because it included not only the attempt to better oneself, but also a desire to do so by surpassing others. Later, he came to see the interpersonally competitive aspect of this model as more neurotic than primary, and finally identified the "striving for perfection" as the thrust of human development and personality. It is the desire to achieve all of one's potential, to approach his or her ideal state of being and achievement.

This model contains a revolutionary implication. Freud's model was able to explain all current thought, affect, and behavior on the basis of inborn biology and past experience. Adler's schema maintains that people are driven by potential; therefore the future, not just the past, also shapes the present. This teleological approach substantially weakens the imperative of psychic determinism. Changing one's goals and ideals has an influence on the present. We will deal below with the ramifications of this philosophy on pathogenesis and treatment.

FICTIONS

In the Introduction, we acknowledged that the theories we describe cannot be truths. Rather, we adopt certain beliefs because they help us make sense of things. Adler applied this principle to everyday living as well. Most people get up in the morning convinced they will survive the day and get up the next morning, even though there is no proof of such an outcome. Many people organize their thinking and behavior around notions of good and evil, for which there can also be no objective proof. Just like the theories of science, such day-to-day beliefs make it possible to function. And, like the theories of science, they shape a person's perceptions and the meaning he or she assigns to events.

Adler called such hypotheses "fictions," not in the sense that they are false, but in recognition of the impossibility of ever proving them. Such fictions are necessary because they maintain the possibility of mental function. The particular fictions held by any individual determine what he or she expects of himself or herself and the world. If, for example, one holds that hard work is always rewarded, it will propel him or her to exert effort in ways that are usually socially and personally profitable. On the other hand, the same belief may lead a person to interpret random misfortune as the outcome of not having worked hard enough.

Since Adler kept a teleological perspective in mind, he identified certain fictions that pertained to one's future. Belief in heaven and hell, or on the other hand a conviction that human mortality is final and complete, are fictions that influence a person's expectations and view of the future. In Adler's terminology, these particular fictions are called "finalisms" because they describe ends. Although the subject of fictional finalisms is in the future, the fictions themselves determine one's interpretations and choices in the present. Superiority, the goal of human striving, is itself a fiction shared by all.

STYLE OF LIFE

In Adler's view, with teleological imperatives to development and with enduring fictions guiding perception and behavior, the straightforward Freudian notion of personality as a self-contained entity shaped by drives and trauma was inadequate. Adler preferred to describe a person's "style of life" (what we would today call "lifestyle"). Style of life is a holistic concept including how one conducts himself or herself, how he or she handles problems and interpersonal relations. One's style of life describes how he or she attempts to achieve superiority.

The essence of one's style is determined usually by about age 5, and is influenced by temperament, inner goal orientation, and environmental forces that either foster or impede these motivators. From this perspective, while acknowledging the overriding importance of individuality, Adler described four basic psychological types:

- The ruling type are aggressive and dominant. They attempt to achieve superiority by attaining personal power, with little regard for those in their way. The most forceful may be brutes or bullies.
- The leaning (or getting) type are dependent people who tend not to be assertive. They rely on others to provide for them and are sensitive to slights or rejection. Such people

are vulnerable to classical neuroses such as anxiety and depression.

- The avoiding type cope by withdrawing. They keep away from other people as much as they can and shun confrontation, even with their own self-expectations. In the extreme, they may be schizoid or psychotic.
- The socially useful type is the only healthy category. These are the people who have sufficient energy to devote to constructive engagement with other human beings. The other three styles of life Adler described as "mistaken" types.

Unlike Freud, who seemed to paint families as faceless and interchangeable, Adler saw some specificity in how early caregivers and circumstances could affect the evolution of style of life. He identified three particular situations that might negatively affect one's lifestyle:

- Organ inferiority, or childhood disease, can leave children feeling burdened and self-centered. They will gravitate toward a leaning or dependent lifestyle, or they may overcompensate and adopt a (shallow and fragile) dominant style. True compensation requires the sensitive attention of parents.
- Pampering or spoiling leaves children with unmodified primitive fantasies of gratification. They come to expect their wishes to be fulfilled by those around them. As the child ventures into the world outside the family, he or she is left without any means of obtaining satisfaction other than demanding it and quickly comes to feel inferior.
- Neglect is the opposite of pampering, but it yields a similar outcome. A neglected child not only comes into the world inferior but learns every day that those closest to him or her confirm that inferiority. Since they cannot learn to trust others, these children become selfish. And since they have no experience receiving love, they are unable to offer it.

SOCIAL INTEREST

A major focus of contention between Adler and Freud was Adler's early and energetic emphasis on the social context of human development, behavior, and pathology. For Adler, social interest was second only to the striving for perfection as a motivating factor. Since he began from a holistic perspective, Adler saw humans as social animals that cannot be separated from their social context. Even striving for perfection is shaped by social norms. And even the most hostile, dominating person can only be hostile or dominating toward other people. Much like style of life, the tendency toward social interest is inborn, but it must be nurtured by the environment. For example, furthering one's own welfare may require the suffering of another. While it is innate human nature to advance oneself at the expense of another, social pressures promote the development of empathic concern. Social interest usually involves some element of self-sacrifice, and the social environment provides rewards for that sacrifice.

Adler was careful to differentiate social interest from social skill or extroversion. Being friendly and demonstrative may be one manifestation of genuine social interest, or it may simply be a vehicle for advancing one's selfish ends. Social interest for Adler meant a broader notion of caring for others: family, community, and society. From this perspective, it is clear why being socially useful was his definition of psychological health.

BIRTH ORDER

While Freud and most of his followers at least acknowledged the influence of parents on development, Adler was probably the first theorist to attend to the role of siblings in shaping personality. His notions of the importance of birth order (whatever may be said for their scientific validity) have demonstrated enduring popularity even among those who have never heard of Alfred Adler. In context, however, even Adler regarded birth order as a useful fiction for understanding people, not a profound truth.

The only child is likely to grow up a pampered one, as described above. Having no rival for his or her parents' affection and attention, the only child comes to expect special care and need not learn to share. On the other hand, the only child of neglectful or abusive parents must bear the burden alone.

The first child begins, of course, as an only child. But when the first sibling arrives, the world changes dramatically. Displaced from the sole position of honor, the first child may attempt to compensate in any of a number of ways. Commonly, children will regress, acting like babies themselves to get what the baby has taken away. This reaction is rarely successful, as most parents will tell him or her to grow up. Some children will respond by becoming defiant and contrary. Others may withdraw and become sullen. Adler thought that first children were more likely to become problem children as they attempted to find ways to compensate for their loss of superiority. On the other hand, he also acknowledged that, in compensation, they were also more likely than others to become precocious. The result, of course, depends on both temperament and upbringing. In general, Adler thought first children were more likely than others to turn out solitary and conservative.

The second child enters the world not only with the inferiority inherent in the human condition, but also with the added shadow of his or her older sibling's obvious superiority. From the beginning, life is a competition—if not with the actual brother or sister, then at least with the internal image of that superior sibling—and quite often remains so. Driven to succeed, many will achieve a good deal, but will often be left with the sense of incomplete achievement. Others will become more withdrawn, and will give up the fight, convinced they cannot win anyway. Subsequent middle children resemble the second child, though each will choose his or her rival in the family.

The youngest child is most likely to be pampered. He or she is never displaced from the coddled position of baby. Like firstborns, youngest children may grow up spoiled and entitled. Or, they may feel even more inferior than middle children, because they never have the experience of superiority to junior siblings. Adler saw youngest children as only slightly less likely than firstborns to create problems. They may be driven by their perceived inferiority to become either dependent or reactively dominant. As always, there is the opportunity for healthy channeling of these tendencies, and youngest children can develop a healthy drive to succeed and a strong social interest.

PSYCHOPATHOLOGY

From our survey of Adler's theories of development and function, it is a short step to outline what can go wrong. Since psychological life is primarily a striving for perfection or superiority, and since social interest is inherent in the very definition of a healthy lifestyle, disruptive influences on either of these threads will result in pathological outcomes. Necessarily, pathology is characterized by inferiority and lack of social interest.

A person who feels competent and confident, one with a solid foundation of superiority, can afford to direct energy toward others. But those who are burdened by inferiority are desperately focusing attention on themselves. Adler, as we have seen, acknowledged many normative sources of inferiority, for example: bodily imperfections, birth order, and parental failings. Ideally, people make up for these inferiorities. The small, weak child may devote himself or herself to exercise and physical improvement, or may pursue intellectual or artistic sources of superiority. Adler noted that most of the games and toys of children are an effort to emulate adults; they are normal ways of striving for perfection and superiority in the face of childhood's inherent inferiority.

It is not just people's bodies and families that influence their susceptibility to inferiority. Since we are guided by our fictions, we are vulnerable to their expectations and ideals. One who maintains a fiction that only perfect performance can yield happiness will find himself or herself subject to abundant opportunities to perceive failure and inferiority. Even fictions that are not inherently grossly unrealistic can be problematic, because one's fictions should correlate with one's capacities and lifestyle. A shy and withdrawn person will be repeatedly defeated by a fiction that social success is necessary for happiness. Thus, a mismatch of fictions with reality and/or style of life is a major source of unhappiness.

Adler identified the core of neurotic unhappiness with the now-famous phrase *inferiority complex*. More than just a symptom, the inferiority complex is a pervasive way of interpreting, evaluating, and responding to experience. It is a way of living. Thinking and behavior are molded to be consistent with the tenets of the inferiority complex. In its unmodified manifestations, it is evident as shyness, submission, over-compliance, and neediness. In a real society, such behavior earns at least isolation, if not overt hostility, and leaves the person feeling even more inferior.

In the ideal situation, one compensates for inferiority by developing complementary abilities and/or adjusting one's fictions. A more neurotic adaptation is the development of the *superiority complex*. Adler saw inferiority at the heart of the ruling lifestyle, and that adaptation can assume harmful proportions by pervading every aspect of one's thought and conduct. Attempting to override their own inferiority by subjecting others, these neurotics become bullies and braggarts, insensitive to the feelings of those they hurt, yet unable ever to attain satisfaction themselves. Adler saw addictions as a dimension of this type of pathology, through the chemically induced delusion of superiority.

Since social interest is inherent in psychological health, it follows that lack of social concern is inherent in mental illness. Problem children, suicides, and sociopaths are all psychological failures because they lack social interest. Their goal remains fixed as one of personal superiority, and they have nothing left to offer society.

MR. BROWN exhibits a typical inferiority complex. He is having a difficult time achieving a sense of superiority in almost any realm. His behavior is common for second children. Feeling inferior to his accomplished older brother, he continues to see the same sibling rivalry in school and work. Unconsciously convinced he is perpetually doomed to lose the struggles, he manages by neurotic maneuvers to withdraw from them. Mr. Brown has adopted a lifestyle primarily of the avoiding type.

Mr. Brown is caught by his own fiction that he must achieve perfection to win the competition. Since he is aware of being at least imperfect, he experiences every echo of sibling rivalry as a confrontation of immense consequence. Because of his sense of inferiority, he is unable to invest energy in the healthy pursuit of social interest. As a result, his connections to family and work suffer.

TECHNICAL IMPLICATIONS

More interested in the theory and philosophy of his work than in its clinical ramifications, Adler wrote little about technique; but he did write some, and other conclusions are obvious from his intent. Since maladaptive fictions underlie so much pathology, Adler would begin by identifying these and their sources. He paid significant attention to birth order and to childhood illnesses or injuries. Like Freud, he looked at earliest memories, not as descriptions of historic truths, but as indicators of models for current lifestyle. He would particularly investigate a patient's upbringing: what behaviors were encouraged or inhibited and by what means. Also, like Freud (and Jung, as we will see later in this chapter), Adler attended to dreams, but his interpretations were relatively direct. He saw the content of dreams as reflective of the dreamer's style of life and of his or her guiding fictions. And unlike Freud, who regarded external events as interchangeable triggers for neurotic responses, Adler attributed specific import to influential events such as losses or social pressures.

If his theory split Adler from Freud, his therapeutic implementation of it constituted an irreconcilable rift. Adler went to great lengths to avoid the authoritarian trappings that were necessary for Freud's nurturance of transference. He saw any effort on the patient's part to endow the analyst with authority as a replay of his or her pathological style of coping with inferiority— by leaning dependently or by setting up failures in the hopes of establishing neurotic superiority. Where Freud would see a patient's resistance to therapy or personal change as a matter of enforcing repression, Adler saw it as a failure of courage to give up the neurotic lifestyle.

Adler abandoned the couch and sat face to face with his patients, thereby encouraging them to be partners in their own growth. By focusing on repeated examples of the intrusion of fictions and lifestyle into the patient's search for happiness, Adler would encourage modifications of both. And since he saw social interest as necessary for growth, he would encourage thinking and behavior in the direction of increasing social interest, often with direct suggestions and recommendations. It is in this domain that he would make use of the transference. By forming a productive and meaningful relationship with the analyst, the patient gains the experience of a positive social encounter and can transfer this learning to other aspects of his or her life.

Carl Jung

A more radical dissent from the Freudian mainstream came from the man to whom Freud once wished to pass the mantle of psychoanalytic authority, Carl Jung (1875–1961). Jung was born in rural Switzerland to a Protestant parson. His father began teaching him Latin at age 6, and he developed a lifelong interest in languages. Besides being fluent in many modern European tongues, he learned ancient ones including Sanskrit, the original language of Hindu writings. A solitary youngster, he buried himself in studies and devoted much of his energy to the mystical and heavily symbolic traditions of alchemy, kaballah, gnosticism, Hinduism, and Buddhism.

Although he wished to study archaeology, he was persuaded that medicine was a more practical pursuit. Under the influence of the famous neurologist Krafft-Ebing at the University of Basel, Jung chose a career in psychiatry. His first position, at the Burghöltzi Mental Hospital in Zurich, exposed him to Eugen Bleuler, the man who first described, and named, schizophrenia. He read and admired Freud's works and met him in 1907. Legend has it that, on that first encounter, Freud was so taken with Jung that he canceled his appointments for the rest of the day, and that the two of them talked for 13 hours straight. Freud was not only smitten with Jung's intellect and creativity, he also saw cultural and political reasons to mentor the young Swiss analyst. The circle of followers around Freud was almost exclusively Viennese and predominantly Jewish, and they were attempting to promulgate a theory that shocked or offended many with its emphasis on the unconscious and on sexual drives. Jung, as a Swiss Protestant, could bring a more universal appeal to the psychoanalytic movement; Freud hoped and planned that Jung would be his heir as the leader of psychoanalytic thought. Jung became the first president of the International Psychoanalytic Society and accompanied Freud on a trip to lecture at Clark University in Massachusetts in 1909.

Ideological differences, however, would prove insurmountable. Jung never completely subscribed to the limits of drive theory, and Freud could not accept the cultural and mystical dimensions of Jung's thinking. During their transatlantic lecture trip, the two were analyzing each other's dreams. Their disagreements grew so emotional that their bond was severely strained. By 1913, the two had completely renounced each other.

Jung had always possessed a capacity for very lucid dreaming. In 1913, he had a "vision" of a flood engulfing Europe, drowning thousands of people and their civilization. There followed weeks of dreams about floods, blood, and death. Jung was afraid he was going insane, but with the subsequent outbreak of World War I, he felt he had tapped into a potent dimension of his unconscious, one which would provide the heartbeat for much of the rest of his work. He would come to see Freud's unconscious as a very small playground of the human mind and soul and would elaborate perhaps the most colorful of all theories of personality.

STRUCTURE

Jung saw the psyche consisting of three parts. Although some of the terms are the same as Freud's, the meanings are different.

- *Ego* is the conscious mind. It includes all of one's capacity to think, feel, and remember, and correlates roughly with Freud's system Cs from the topographic model.
- *Personal unconscious* contains both accessible memories and those that have become repressed. It resembles Freud's systems UCs and PCs, but specifically does not include the drives and instincts of the Freudian model. Experiences in the personal unconscious are groped into clusters Jung called "complexes" (which have nothing to do with Adler's superiority and inferiority complexes). A complex is an organized group of thoughts and feelings about a particular concept, sometimes around a particular object. Jung often cited the example of the mother complex, a collection of emotions, ideas, and recollections around one's own experience of being mothered. Complexes have the power of "constellation," the ability to draw in new experiences and incorporate them. Thus an experience with a nurturing teacher may be added to the mother complex and modify it.
- *Collective unconscious* is the feature entirely novel with Jung. It is a collection of potentials that all humans share, the knowledge with which we are all born. The collective unconscious is the transpersonal element of the human psyche.

  Unlike the personal unconscious, the collective unconscious can never be directly known. It can only be identified indirectly by the influences it exerts, particularly on the emotions. Falling in love with the perfect other, feeling elevated by a work of art, recognizing the meaning of common myths; these are all ways in which the collective unconscious makes its presence known. Where Freud saw myths as symbolic representations of the innate drives, Jung saw the myths as deeper shared inheritances, and the drive manifestations as smaller contemporary effects of the deeper recollections.

Archetypes

The collective unconscious is populated by entities called *archetypes*. (On some occasions, Jung called them *imagos* or *dominants*.) The archetype is an inborn tendency to sense things in a certain way. It has no inherent form of its own, but acts as an organizing influence that shapes and gives meaning to human perception and experience. In Freud's scheme, the infant is born with drives and objects are assembled as they relate to the drives. In Jung's, people and history accumulate meaning as they relate to the archetypes. The archetype is thus described by the experiences it draws to itself. Where the drives' demands are biological, those of the archetypes are spiritual.

Just as the personal unconscious is organized around complexes, the collective unconscious is organized around archetypes. We illustrated the mother complex above; there is also a mother archetype. People are born with an ability to recognize the experience of being mothered. Expectably, one projects that archetype onto elements of the world, most particularly onto his or her real mother. Whether or not such a person is available, people will personify the archetype in cultural and mythological images. In Western culture, Eve and Mary are typical examples; more broadly, a clinic, one's country, or nature can serve that function.

The family also serves as basis for other archetypes. The father archetype may be symbolized by a figure of guidance or authority. The child archetype is celebrated in myth and religion.

While there is no fixed number or list of archetypes, many are common. The hero shows up in cultures ancient and modern. The maiden represents purity and innocence. The wise old man appears often. The trickster frequently wears the guise of magician or clown. Archetypes can also be animals, such as the snake and the falcon.

For Jung, even the self is an archetype. Two other important pairs of archetypes, persona and shadow, and anima and animus, are elaborated later in this chapter, but require first a detour through Jung's theories of personality.

ATTITUDES AND FUNCTIONS

Jung had little use for Freud's dynamic model of mental function. He was more interested in how the mind allocates and uses psychic energy and how it orients itself to the world. His system rests on three dynamic principles:

- *The principle of opposites*—Everything immediately suggests its opposite. It is impossible to have a good thought without an accompanying bad thought, because without the concept of bad, it is impossible to define good, and vice versa. Without negative and positive poles, a battery can generate no energy.
- *The principle of equivalence*—The energy of opposition is equally divided between both sides of the contrast. A strong sense of love will arouse a strong sense of hate; a weak feeling of amusement will engender a weak sense of irritation. If a person is aware of his or her negative feelings, then the energy associated with them is redirected toward growth of the self; if not, the energy becomes invested in complexes that divert one from growth. These complexes are represented in the "shadow," which will be defined later in this chapter.
- *The principle of entropy*—In physics, energy inherently becomes more disorganized. Heat initiating in a candle becomes evenly distributed in its surroundings. For Jung, opposites become less divided as one ages, and the total energy invested in these contrasts decreases. Polar oppositions of ideas and feelings, invested with great energy in adolescence, are held with much more equanimity in middle age.

Jung described essential typologies of human personality grounded in two attitudes and four functions. The attitudes define how and where one turns for energy and satisfaction. *Introversion* is the movement of energy toward one's inner world. Introverts regard their subjective, inner reality as most important. They value their own thoughts, feelings, and fantasies over the external world. *Extroversion* is a preferential interest in the outer world. Extroverts turn to social contact for energy and gratification. Other people and objects are more important than their own inner world.

Both introverts and extroverts have preferred ways of dealing with the world. Jung described four ways of doing so, which he termed *functions*:

- *Sensing* is the accumulation of information through the senses. A sensing person prefers to relate to the world by looking, listening, and learning. Sensing is perception without judgment.
- *Thinking* is the evaluation of ideas or information using logic and reason. It includes judgment and decision making.
- *Feeling* is also a way of evaluating information, but uses emotion. Jung meant it to include the totality of affective response to an idea or perception.
- *Intuition* is a mode of perception that operates outside usual consciousness. It involves a response to personal signals that cannot be as readily identified as senses or emotions. Jung compared it to "seeing around corners."

Each function is present to some extent in every individual, and ideally one should seek to develop them all. But each person

TABLE 2-1 | *Jung's Typologies*

		Extroversion	Introversion
Superior function	Sensing	Seeks pleasure and new experiences. Reality-oriented, represses intuition.	Passive and calm. Artistic, represses intuition.
	Thinking	Prefers fixed rules, represses feelings. Tries to be objective, may be dogmatic.	Private, theoretical, intellectual. Represses feelings, avoids interpersonal difficulties.
	Feeling	Sociable, emotional, represses thinking. Seeks to connect to the world, respects tradition and authority.	Quiet, thoughtful, hypersensitive. Represses thinking. May seem indifferent to others.
	Intuition	Creative, enjoys new ideas. Bases decisions on hunches. Seeks to connect to unconscious wisdom, represses sensing.	Mystical, dreamy. Embraces unusual ideas, represses sensing. Seldom understood by others.

has one *superior* function; others are less well developed. The combination of introverted or extroverted attitude with the most prominent function determines one's character type. The typologies sort out as illustrated in Table 2-1. Jung described himself as an intuitive introvert. (Contemporary readers may recognize these typologies from their similarity to the classifications of the Myers Briggs Type Indicator, a popular instrument closely derived from Jung's schema.)

INTERPLAY OF OPPOSITES

It is evident that the attitudes and functions cluster into pairs of opposite or complementary tendencies: introversion and extroversion, feeling and thinking, sensing and intuition. The archetypes, too, include lovers and warriors, gods and demons. While the ideal person would be fully in touch with all these capacities, most human beings are incapable of doing so. Repression serves to sort out what is closest to consciousness. The result is a division into two distinct archetypes:

- *Persona* (from the Greek for "mask") is the social role one assumes. It represents a compromise between one's true (though often unknown) identity and one's social face. Persona begins as an archetype, the image of a socially acceptable person. Repeated social encounters, modifications, and deliberate alterations eventually bring the persona far from the stream of the collective unconscious. At its most benign, the persona consists of that face necessary to do one's business in the world and make connections, often psychologically and spiritually profitable ones. But it can also be used to manipulate for less productive purposes. The danger arises when the individual believes his or her persona is the true self.
- *Shadow* is what is repressed from the most ancient elements of the collective unconscious, the animal parts of the self. It contains the brutal capabilities of human nature: selfishness, hate, and violence. Human animals can never be free of such motives. The difference in their effect is in how far removed they are from awareness. Shadow also contains the repressed elements of attitude and function (e.g., the thinking capability in a primarily feeling person). As in all of Jung's dualities, awareness is associated with health,

and one who keeps these urges totally unrecognized will suffer from them in dreams, in personal distress, and in social conflict.

Another dichotomy addressed by Jung is that of sex roles. One's role as man or woman is part of the persona. Like Freud, Jung believed that humans are in the beginning bisexual, and that sex roles differentiate with development. Biology and society are the major determinants of outward expression and conscious identity. But the tendency towards the opposite sex is contained in two particular archetypes:

- *Anima* is the feminine side of the male psyche. It is emotional, nurturing, and connected to life forces. Images of the anima include the earth mother, the witch, or the intuitive young girl.
- *Animus* is the masculine side of the female psyche. It emphasizes rational thought and accomplishment. Symbols include the sorcerer, the sage, and the general.

Jung was probably even more rigid than Freud in his belief in the difference between the psychologies of men and women: Women are characterized by their abilities to enter relationships; men, by their abilities to engage in reason and analysis. But in this dichotomy again, he saw balance as critical. Awareness of the opposite tendency helps one relate to the other sex, which is both a biological and a psychological necessity. The combination of anima and animus in each person is called *szyzygy*. From Jung's perspective, falling in love is a search for one's missing other half.

Self plays a unique role in Jung's theory. For him, the self is not simply a psychological construct, it is an archetype. It represents the unification of all the opposing tendencies and abilities. The self is both introverted and extroverted, sensing and intuitive, masculine and feminine. It straddles the boundaries between conscious and unconscious, between rational and irrational. The self draws in and harmonizes archetypes and their expressions. It allocates psychic energy appropriate for each end and its setting. Thus, the self, not the ego, is the true center of the Jungian personality.

The development of the self is the ultimate goal of psychological development. However, the achievement of this type of balance requires the full development of its component capacities. Energy must first be directed toward defining one's characteristics and negotiating with the world before it can be redirected toward the balance of opposites. Therefore, self-realization is usually not achieved before middle age. By then, the development of self ultimately makes one less self-centered.

TECHNICAL IMPLICATIONS

Jung eschewed any diagnostic system based on symptoms or behavior. He did not name diseases or syndromes. In simplest terms, he regarded all troubles of the human psyche as failures on the road to self-realization. These defects generally resulted from the failure to recognize or integrate attitudes, functions, tendencies, or capacities. His aim in therapy was to bring those neglected aspects into the light and promote their unfolding. He divided analysis into four stages, never clearly differentiated in time or sequence:

1. *Confession* is the stage where one relates his or her story to the analyst. More than just history, it includes the cathartic exposure of one's guilts, fears, and regrets. For Jung, this stage first allows the analysand to relieve himself or herself of much of the burden by sharing it, and also begins to allow him or her to make contact with the shadow.

2. *Elucidation* is comparable to Freud's process of interpretation. Symptoms and behavior are examined through the filter of failed development of attitude or function and for subversions of the demands of archetypes. Here Jung would listen for manifestations of the collective unconscious.

3. *Education* involves using the confessed and elucidated material and examining parallels in myth and literature. Doing so often highlights the guiding fictions of one's life. A major benefit of this process is to allow the patient to see and feel himself or herself as a vital part of the human species, sharing common dreams and history.

4. *Transformation* occurs when one confronts the many repressed and neglected parts that have been brought into awareness. Jung and his followers used many methodical and concrete techniques in this phase. Patients were instructed to record dreams and associations, to accumulate symbols related to their dreams, thoughts, and feelings.

They would be encouraged to draw or make models of these images and would be directed to the library to seek literary and mythological connections. By making concrete connections to civilization's enduring symbols, the person can transcend the limited self and connect to the greater whole of humanity.

Jung himself compared analysis to alchemy. It relies heavily on intuition, and carries considerable faith in powers and processes inaccessible to the mind of either patient or analyst. The end he sought was nowhere close to Freud's relief of neurotic symptoms. He wanted to bring his patients to health by guiding them to a transcendent connection with human experience and history.

Learning points

- In Alfred Adler's model, people are guided unconsciously by a number of fictions. Chief among these is the search for superiority. A mismatch between one's fictions and his or her capabilities or environment yields psychological distress.
- A person's style of life describes how he or she attempts to achieve superiority or perfection. Style of life is based on both temperament and environment. The four basic styles are: ruling, leaning, avoiding, and socially useful; the last is the only fully healthy lifestyle.
- Social interest is the highest motivator of healthy human activity for Adler.
- Adler elaborated characteristics based on birth order:
  - Firstborns tend to be high achievers and may be domineering.
  - Middle children may become passive and disappear, or may attempt to overachieve.
  - Youngest children tend to be pampered and self-centered.
- Carl Jung drew attention to the collective unconscious, the inborn memory of human civilization.
- The collective unconscious manifests itself in multiple archetypes, organizing influences manifest in myth and symbol.

- Jung described two major attitudes (introversion and extroversion) and four functions (sensing, thinking, feeling, and intuition). Together, the attitudes and functions define eight typologies of personality.
- Self-realization is the aim of human development and requires the integration of opposite tendencies and capacities within the mind and spirit.

RECOMMENDED READINGS

Allen BP. *Personality Theories: Development, Growth, and Diversity.* 2nd ed. Boston: Allyn and Bacon, 1997.

Boeree CG. *Personality Theories.* [Electronic textbook on Shippensburg University Web site] Available at: http://www.ship.edu/~cgboeree/perscontents.html. Accessed April 28, 2005.

Engler B. *Personality Theories.* 5th ed. Boston: Houghton Mifflin Co., 1999.

Stevens A. *An Intelligent Person's Guide to Psychotherapy.* London: Duckworth and Co., 1998.

Sweeny TJ. *Adlerian Counseling: A Practitioner's Approach.* Philadelphia: Accelerated Development, 1998.

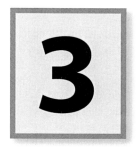

Ego Psychology

"Mind is the great lever of all things; human thought is the process by which human ends are ultimately answered."
—Daniel Webster

LEARNING OBJECTIVES

The reader will be able to:

1. Define the major defense mechanisms.
2. Describe the process and significance of adaptation.
3. Outline the ego psychological perspective of the origin of the psychic structures.

EGO AND DEFENSE MECHANISMS

It is Sigmund Freud's daughter Anna Freud (1895–1982) who is often identified as the first voice of ego psychology. Encouraged by her father to extend the study and practice of psychoanalysis to children, she is best known for elucidating the defense mechanisms by which the ego masters the environment and the shaping forces of each individual's psychopathology, the id and the superego. The names and definitions she assigned are still the benchmark terminology of psychoanalytic psychology: repression, suppression, denial, reaction formation, undoing, rational-

49

ization, intellectualization, sublimation, displacement, and several others. These mechanisms are defined and illustrated in Table 3-1.

Sigmund Freud maintained that repression was the predominant defense mechanism, that it was the chief tool available to the ego to defend itself against the environment and the impulses of the id. The major thrust of analysis, therefore, was to uncover and comprehend the content of the repressed material. Anna Freud's articulation of the richness of the defense mechanisms pointed analysts toward the examination of the dynamic processes operative within the ego itself. However, she maintained that analysis of the ego paled by comparison with analysis of the id.

MR. BROWN has *repressed* his envy of his brother and his resentment of his father. He has *identified with the aggressor* by adopting his father's line of work. His superego, however, makes him feel guilty about having succeeded in his Oedipal strivings for closeness with his mother, and his failures at work and school represent self-punishment.

ADAPTATION AND DIFFERENTIATION

The promulgation of ego psychological theory fell to a generation of analysts who were mostly refugees from Hitler's advance through Europe, and who had to postpone their major work until they could resettle in the 1930s. These included Ernst Kris, Rudolph Lowenstein, Rene Spitz, and chief among Freud's protégés, Heinz Hartmann (1894–1970). A trainee of Freud's, Hartmann undertook the expansion of his mentor's model to explain some of its lingering questions: What was the origin of ego? How did ego tame id, which was powered by the potent energy of the drives? What was the purpose of the aggressive drive? What role did these structures and forces play in normal development?

For Hartmann, the unifying process of human psychological development was adaptation, a reciprocal relationship between the individual and his or her environment. The outcome of successful adaptation is a "fitting together" of the individual with the environment. Thus, conflict is neither the cause nor the outcome of psychopathology, but a normal and necessary part of the human

TABLE 3-1	Ego Defense Mechanisms Elaborated by Anna Freud	
Mechanism	**Definition**	**Example**
Repression	Involuntary exclusion from conscious awareness of conflictual or painful impulses, thoughts, or memories	Battered child has no memories from before age 7.
Suppression	Conscious exclusion from awareness of painful impulses, thoughts, or memories	"I choose not to think about that."
Denial	Failure to recognize external reality	Patient with malignant tumor insists she does not have cancer.
Reaction formation	Reversal of an impulse to its opposite	Jealous older sister becomes very affectionate and protective of newborn brother.
Undoing	Symbolic or actual negation of previous unacceptable thought or action	Woman has fleeting thought of killing her husband; unaware of it, she brings him a gift that night.
Rationalization	Elaboration of socially acceptable reasons to justify feelings or actions that are unconsciously determined	Embarrassed by his rival's intellectual superiority, boy criticizes the other's nerdy dress.
Intellectualization	Overuse of reasoning or logic to avoid awareness of feelings and impulses	Adolescent talks at great length about social issues to avoid confronting his own aggressive impulses.
Sublimation	Partial gratification of an impulse by altering the aim or object to make it socially more acceptable	Man channels aggressive urges into athletic competition.

(continues)

TABLE 3-1	Ego Defense Mechanisms Elaborated by Anna Freud (continued)	
Mechanism	**Definition**	**Example**
Symbolization	Representation of affect-laden person, thing, or thought in the form of another person, thing, or thought that has some similarity of association	Sometimes a cigar isn't just a cigar. . . .
Somatization	Expression of psychic conflict by production of physical symptom, sometimes symbolic of the conflict	Afraid of being bullied at school, child develops a stomachache.
Displacement	Affect originally attached to one object is transferred to a more innocuous object	Man is embarrassed and angry for being criticized by boss at work; ashamed of his powerlessness to object in public he comes home and kicks the dog.
Aim inhibition	Accepting partial gratification of an impulse	Man cultivates close friendship with woman who is sexually desired but socially forbidden to him.
Introjection (or internalization)	Assimilation of characteristics of an object into one's own ego/superego	Man envies his boss, so he adopts his politics and tastes.
Identification	Modeling of one's self on another person or group, but with less intensity and completeness than with introjection	Conscious emulation of an admired public figure.
Identification with the aggressor	Incorporation of aspects of another person who is perceived as a serious threat or cause of frustration	Boy in Oedipal stage assumes characteristics of father.

(continues)

TABLE 3-1	Ego Defense Mechanisms Elaborated by Anna Freud (continued)	

Mechanism	Definition	Example
Idealization	Overestimation of positive and underestimation of negative qualities of a desired object	Widower is unable to recall any of the things he ever resented about his wife.
Projection	Attributing one's own unacknowledged feelings and impulses to another person	Woman represses her own sexual hunger and dismisses all men as sex fiends.
Regression	Return to previous level of function or psychosexual stage	Five-year-old boy resumes bedwetting when sibling is born.
Splitting	Perceiving of objects as all good or all bad	Man can have sex with prostitutes but must treat wife as a chaste saint.
Dissociation	Splitting off of a group of thoughts or actions from conscious awareness	Fugue state.
Isolation (of affect)	Repression of affect away from a thought, or a thought away from its affect	Medical student dissects cadaver without any feelings about death.
Fantasy	Mental elaborations that provide partial gratification of impulses	Man with erectile dysfunction daydreams about orgies.
Turning (aggression) against the self	Self-destructive thoughts or actions replace aggression toward other objects	Woman blocks anxiety over fight with husband by getting into minor auto accident.
Turning passive into active	Action in anticipation of being acted upon	Patient misses therapy session just before therapist's announced vacation.

condition. In Hartmann's model, the ingredients of ego and id are present at birth in an undifferentiated matrix. Normative conflicts with the environment separate ego from id. Particularly, the infant expectably experiences certain degrees of frustration, as his or her too-human mother fails to provide total and immediate satisfaction. In fact, if there remained total gratification, there would never be any need to differentiate self from other, to pursue autonomy; in short, no need for an ego.

Id, ego, and superego continue to separate by the process of *differentiation*. Within the ego, primitive regulatory factors are increasingly replaced or supplemented by more effective ones. The experiences of frustration, in the context of normative growth of brain and body, allow the developing ego to remember experiences long enough to delay gratification and anticipate the future. Part of the power the ego derives from the gradually differentiating matrix serves to gratify id desires, though not in the immediate and unrestrained terms of the primitive mind. In a reciprocal fashion, the memory of past gratification allows the ego to engage in delayed gratification. This process mandates the creation of an internal world of object representations; and this inner world facilitates further exercise of delayed gratification. As the structures ego and superego mature, the need for external fulfillment diminishes and autonomy increases.

Because psychic structures enable the individual to be less dependent on the environment, structure formation serves adaptation. Superego is one outcome of adaptation to the social environment, a product of continuing ego development. While ego development depends on the maturation of body and brain to provide motor and cognitive control, superego development is more purely social and abstract. Although Hartmann did not reject castration anxiety as critical in superego development, he placed much more emphasis on identification and idealization. The infant first identifies with his or her parents as idealized figures who provide protection and gratification. Soon he or she discovers that fitting together is better served by some restraint of id urges and by modeling of the moral standards of the parents. These functions constitute the role of the superego. (See Figure 3-1.)

In drive theory, the drives shape and guide the structures. In ego psychology, the relationship is more complementary. Ego and superego divert libidinal energy away from purely sexual aims by means of sublimation and other mechanisms. Whereas primitive

Sigmund Freud's Model

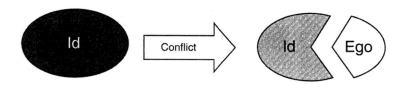

Heinz Hartmann's Model

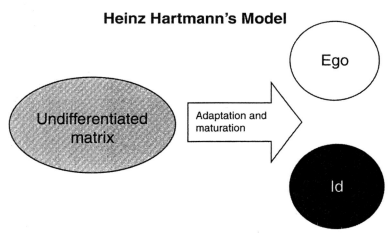

FIGURE 3-1 ▦ Models of the Origin of the Ego.

libido aimed just for erotic gratification, the maturing ego could seek affection, entertainment, and enlightenment. Similarly, aggression is redirected from the desire for destruction of others and is internalized to serve ego. Its power is used by superego to restrain destructive pursuit of id impulses; it is lassoed by ego and transformed into competitiveness and other more adaptive manifestations. Modification of innate aggression proceeds by several means:

▦ Displacement—Aggression is redirected to more acceptable objects such as criminals or the rival soccer team.

- Sublimation—Aggression is completely divorced from an obvious object and diverted to an acceptable aim; energy may be exerted chopping trees or hauling trash.
- Fusion with libido—Healthy adult relationships include both pulling together and pushing apart and ideally the libidinal element predominates. Satisfying sex may include some teasing; an admiring relationship with a mentor may involve competition.

Evolution of Defense Mechanisms

Defense mechanisms are tools for adaptation to the environment by either *alloplastic* means (changing the environment) or *autoplastic* ones (changing the self). Alloplastic solutions require the cooperation or subservience of elements outside the self and are thus often thwarted. The mature, confident ego is more apt to attempt autoplastic solutions, which are more likely to be successful. The child who persists in demanding attention from an unresponsive parent is certain to be frustrated. If he or she learns to entertain himself or herself and to find pleasure in friends, gratification is at hand.

In the earliest stages of ego development, the role of the defenses is to minimize pain and distress and to gratify id wishes. Later, they serve to contain and master id's conflicts with reality and with superego. Eventually, though, many applications of the defense mechanisms lose their purely defensive function. The mechanisms that began as reflexes can come to change personality.

Identification is the principle example, though hardly the only one. As noted above, in the infant, identification protects against the powerlessness of being a victim of one's environment. Later, it promotes the development of superego function. In the social realm, the child who identifies with his or her peers learns how to blend into the group and achieves the libidinal gratification of belonging. But even at this early stage, identification achieves its own rewards independent of defensive purpose. Identifying with an admired teacher promotes the development of intellectual or artistic skills that provide satisfaction outside the context of drive gratification or defense against distress. This transformation of ego functions outside the defensive realm allows ego psychology to explain nuances of personality development with a richness not available to drive psychology.

MS. GRAY learned early from identification with her mother that sexual behavior could bring some form of intimacy and support from men. As an adult, she is able to attract men easily. At times, she does so to defend against loneliness, but at other times she can mobilize this capacity to provide entertainment and even fulfillment. Even while intellectually aware of its destructive consequences, she identifies this aptitude with some pride as part of her self-definition.

There is also a *conflict-free sphere* of ego development. Certain capacities have an inherent capacity for expression and growth, promoting adaptation to the environment without need to invoke conflict. Apparatuses that exist within the undifferentiated matrix come under control of the ego. In the motor sphere, these capacities include grasping, crawling, and walking. In the mental realm, they encompass perception, object comprehension, thinking, language, and memory. These faculties, though not defenses, are indispensable for coping and for growth. Their development is fueled by the inherent satisfaction and pleasure the ego gleans by exercising them.

EARLY EGO DEVELOPMENT

Hartmann and his contemporaries described the structure and function of id, ego, and superego and postulated their developmental origins in retrospect. Rene Spitz was a successor to Hartmann and elaborated in more detail the development of ego using direct observations of children.

Spitz began by considering the role of perception in the infant. For the baby, sensation is all visceral and poorly differentiated. Self and other, inside and outside, are initially fused; sensations are poorly discriminated from each other, if at all; experiences are either all good or all bad and very intense. Experience with a partner, usually mother, allows for some modulation of the intensity. Repeated experiences establish memory traces. Interaction with mother allows the child to put these memories to work in the service of the ego; he or she learns to become an agent in his or her world, not just a passive recipient of its gifts or pains. Spitz identified three organizing principles in the development of the ego:

1. The smiling response—Usually at about age 3 months, the child begins to smile in the presence of pleasant stimuli.

The singular perceptual mode of earliest life is replaced by diacritical perception, the earliest separation of inside from outside. Recognition of specific faces is evidence of the establishment of memory traces. The ability to connect the face of the present with the memory of pleasure in the past is the manifestation of an ability to form associations. The rudimentary ego is able to shift from passive and random behaviors to active and directed ones. Here begin social relations.

2. Stranger anxiety—At about 8 months, most children express distress in the presence of unfamiliar people. This feature is possible because the child can now specify the affective connection to the familiar parent. Additionally, anxiety is no longer just an unavoidable response to current distress, but has begun to serve a signal function. Even though the stranger is not inflicting pain or discomfort, the young ego experiences anxiety as a signal that some affliction may be in the offing.

3. Semantic communication—Most children can speak at about 1 year of age, but it is not until about 6 months later that they can formulate words with the specific intent to communicate something to another. One of the earliest ways this function is evident is in the ability to say "no." Doing so, the child takes the first steps in identification with the aggressor, turning passivity into active control. Learning to communicate by speaking, the child comes to relinquish the fantasy of perfect nonverbal communication with a symbiotic partner. In doing so, the child takes his or her first steps toward a full social life.

ADULT DEVELOPMENT

The ego in this psychology was not just a more complex entity than in the drive model, it was also a more vital and organic one, growing and changing even in adult life. Since elements of the environment are critical in the formation of the ego in the first place, it stands to reason that they will continue to exert influence on the ego long after childhood. Two theorists made particularly lasting contributions to the theories of adult development: Erik Erikson and George Vaillant.

TABLE 3-2	Erikson's Stages of Psychosocial Development	
Life Crisis	**Usual Age**	**Summary**
Basic trust vs. basic mistrust	0–1 year	World is a reliable place; I am reliable vs. world is dangerous; I cannot trust myself
Autonomy vs. shame and doubt	1–3 years	I can exert myself and accomplish things vs. I am incompetent and unsuccessful
Initiative vs. guilt	3–6 years	I can follow my curiosity and exploit opportunities vs. It is wrong for me to explore or to initiate
Industry vs. inferiority	6–12 years	I can take pleasure in my achievements vs. I am not as capable as my peers
Identity vs. identity diffusion	Adolescence	I can define myself as an independent person vs. I can only define myself in terms of the expectations of others
Intimacy vs. isolation	Young adulthood	I can achieve emotional closeness with others vs. Getting close is more risky than it is worth
Generativity vs. self-absorption	Middle adulthood	My contributions live on through future generations vs. There is no meaning beyond my finite life
Integrity vs. despair	Late life	I accept what life has dealt me and I accept responsibility for my choices vs. I regret that things were not different, and I fear impending death

Erikson and the Epigenetic Model

Erik Erikson (1902–1994) was an artist and teacher when he met Anna Freud in his mid-20s. Encouraged by her to study psychoanalysis, he became interested in the influence of society and culture on child development. In developing his theories, he did not stop with the evolution of the ego, but elaborated ego's maturation through the span of life. Erikson's definitions of the eight stages of human development have become famous even outside psychodynamic circles. (See Table 3-2.)

From his observations, Erikson posited a succession of life crises, an epigenetic scheme of development:

1. *Basic trust versus basic mistrust*—For the first year of life, the child learns that the world is a trustworthy place and that he or she is also trustworthy. Failure to achieve this end leaves the developing child with a sense of insecurity and an inability to trust others.

2. *Autonomy versus shame and doubt*—From about ages 1 to 3, the developing nervous system affords the opportunity to walk, retain feces, and exert all sorts of self-control. The child can practice leaving mother and returning. But these attempts are not always successful, and failures can lead to self-doubt and shame.

3. *Initiative versus guilt*—From about ages 3 to 6, the growing child attempts to exert influence and follow the leads of curiosity, using his or her budding cognitive and motor skills. The social environment is, however, becoming increasingly important, and when the child violates rules, he or she may feel guilt about the transgression. Of course, this life crisis is exactly contemporary with Freud's Oedipal period. The desire to possess mother and to annihilate father are manifestations of initiative, and the superego, born at this time, is the structural container for guilt. Erikson redefines the essential dynamics of the Oedipal drama to put a greater focus on the role of the social environment.

4. *Industry versus inferiority*—During the latency years, about ages 6 to 12, the child is turning away from parents and toward peers as objects of identification. He or she will seek to excel at sports, school, or other childhood endeavors. The reward is the satisfaction of accomplishment and success. The risk is failure; the child who is benched at softball or who scores a "C" on a math test may learn to feel inferior.

5. *Identity versus identity diffusion*—During puberty and adolescence, the teen is asking, "Who am I?" and constantly revising the answer. A common solution during these years is to assert one's independence by acting, dressing, and talking like everyone else in one's peer group. Identification is an important tool for establishing identity, but it raises the threat of diffusing that sense of individuality.

6. *Intimacy versus isolation*—In young adulthood, the task is to attain a sense of emotional, sexual, and spiritual maturity with a view toward social responsibility. But intimacy carries risks. People are often hurt in trying to establish closeness with others, and if they fail to adapt successfully, they may be inclined to retreat into emotional isolation.

7. *Generativity versus self-absorption*—Middle age is marked by a different kind of questioning, centering on one's place in the larger scheme of life. Generativity is a sense of living on through succeeding generations without becoming overly involved. At the opposite pole is a view that one's life is completely self-contained and finite. Most often, this crisis is played out in raising one's children, but generativity can be accomplished through philanthropy, teaching, entrepreneurship, or other avenues.

8. *Integrity versus despair*—In the closing phase of life, one ideally comes to a sense of balance between owning responsibility for his or her choices and accepting the fate that one has been dealt. Erkison's descriptions of integrity, drawn from observations across cultures, render a richly textured view of spiritual connections with past and future. The task of achieving this goal is daunting and one is threatened with a sense of futility and isolation in the face of impending mortality.

Erikson's model takes ego psychology's basic tenet of adaptation and expands it in the realm of the social environment. It also adds a longitudinal dimension, making for a more flexible, organic map of human development. Some noteworthy features of the epigenetic scheme further amplify its explanatory power:

- No crisis is resolved completely in one direction or the other. An adult who lacks any sense of mistrust would be easily exploited. One who lacks any guilt could be sociopathic. The balance between the poles of any life crisis is a central element of individual personality.
- Crises persist beyond their most relevant phases. Initiative versus guilt, for example, is the signal crisis of the Oedipal period, but adults frequently struggle with issues along the same axis. At each stage, one is still juggling remnants of previous crises.

▨ The resolution of each crisis depends powerfully on the interpersonal environment. The infant who is not fed when hungry cannot learn basic trust. Betrayal by a cherished lover will impair a young adult's capacity to develop intimacy. A society that ridicules elders makes it hard for one to achieve integrity.

 MS. WHITE was raised in an environment that fostered a strong sense of basic trust. Elements of her history indicate that she achieved most of the elements of autonomy, initiative, and industry fairly well. Her current stage of midlife is the time for the struggle of generativity versus self-absorption, and she is indeed striving to define the most adaptive way to be a mother without submerging her own identity. In the midst of this struggle, issues of identity and intimacy, which had previously been negotiated, return in her social withdrawal and her confusion about how to relate to her husband.

MATURATION OF DEFENSES

Erikson's model popularized the notion that psychological development is a lifelong process. His scheme drew on the existing principles of ego psychology, augmented with observations of children and adults in different cultures. A complementary model was developed by George Vaillant (1934–), who examined the patterns of defense mechanisms employed over the lifespan. His methodology was notable. He followed a sizable cohort of healthy young adult men over decades from their 20s into late adulthood and interviewed them in depth to determine what defense mechanisms they employed most commonly and what the consequences were of different patterns of defense.

From his observations, he clustered the defense mechanisms according to the stages of life at which they were most appropriately or most adaptively employed:

▨ Immature defenses include projection, passive aggression, acting out, hypochondriasis, and retreat into fantasy. These defenses are normative in early life. In adulthood, they are characteristic of many personality disorders.

▨ Intermediate (or neurotic) defenses include dissociation, displacement, isolation of affect, intellectualization, repression, and reaction formation. They are common in middle childhood and adolescence. In adulthood, they are most commonly employed in moderately disabling conditions such as generalized anxiety disorder, simple phobias, and dysthymic disorder.

- Mature defenses, characteristic of healthy adults, include altruism, sublimation, anticipation, and humor.

Vaillant's contributions were twofold. First, he undertook an empirical investigation of the evolution of ego function that returned results consistent with the predictions of the prevailing theory. Second, he integrated the cross-sectional descriptions of the defenses that had been used since Freud's time with the longitudinal perspective of Erikson and others.

REFINEMENT OF THE THEORIES

In Freud's formulation, the original psychic structure was id alone. From id's attempts to master the environment, and from the conflicts deriving therefrom, ego arose, at the expense of id strength and energy. In this model, id's drive demands were the source of all mental activity. It explained much, particularly the neurotic symptoms of the patients the early analysts saw. But it failed to account for functions later noted in direct observation of normal children, and it required great logical stretches to explain the problems of patients with more pervasive distortions of perception and response.

Hartmann, noting that elements of ego function, such as perception, were present at birth, postulated instead the undifferentiated matrix. Through both conflict and conflict-free development, ego and id differentiated from the matrix. This model accounted better for what observers were seeing in children, and it provided an internally consistent general philosophy of normal development and function. Additionally, it offered less-tortured interpretations of the more complicated problems that patients brought to analysts as psychoanalysis became a more popular intervention.

Ego psychology used the language of Freud's original drive/structure model and maintained most of its core assumptions. It stretched the explanatory capacities of the model and allowed for the treatment of cases previously impervious to psychoanalysis. Because these patients exhibited more interpersonal problems than strictly intrapsychic ones, and because the model of ego development was contingent on interactions with the personal and social environment, theorists were now presented with a range of questions about the nature of human interaction and its role in development and pathology. The door was opened to schools of thought that described something broader than a one-person psychology. Even while ego psychology was developing further in the 1930s, the schools of interpersonal psychoanalysis and object relations were branching off.

Learning points

- Anna Freud named and described the major psychological defense mechanisms, which are still broadly accepted.
- Heinz Hartmann described psychological development from the perspective of adaptation, the employment of the defense mechanisms to allow the ego to fit together with its environment. Ego psychology focuses on this process as the central element of normal function and psychopathology.
- Ego psychological theory maintains that an undifferentiated matrix of psychic structure is present from birth, and that id, ego, and superego differentiate from it.
- There is a conflict-free sphere of development that encompasses the achievement of capacities such as motor skills and intelligence.
- Ego development continues beyond childhood. Erikson and Vaillant have described the evolution of ego functions throughout life.

RECOMMENDED READINGS

Blanck G, Blanck R. *Ego Psychology: Theory and Practice.* 2nd ed. New York: Columbia University Press, 1994.

Erikson E. *Identity and the Life Cycle: Selected Papers.* New York: International Universities Press, 1959.

Freud A. *The Writings of Anna Freud.* New York: International Universities Press, 1966.

Hartmann H. *Ego Psychology and the Problem of Adaptation.* New York: International Universities Press, 1958.

Polansky N. *Integrated Ego Psychology.* New York: Aldine Pub. Co., 1982.

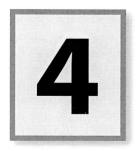

Interpersonal Psychoanalysis

"One realizes that human relationships are the tragic necessity of human life; that they can never be wholly satisfactory, that every ego is half the time greedily seeking them, and half the time pulling away from them. In those simple relationships of loving husband and wife, affectionate sisters, children and grandmother, there are innumerable shades of sweetness and anguish which make up the pattern of our lives day by day."

—Willa Cather

LEARNING OBJECTIVES

The reader will be able to:

1. Define the interpersonal theories of Harry Stack Sullivan.
2. List the neurotic needs identified by Karen Horney.
3. Outline the social psychological theory of Erich Fromm.

As the ego psychologists were delving deeper into the mechanisms of the mind, particularly into its defensive operations and their supporting structures, the society around them was in a state of dramatic turbulence. The social and political movements of the 1920s and 1930s influenced a number of theorists and practitioners. More narrowly, psychoanalysis was discovering the limitations of a one-person psychology. Clinical problems focused less exclusively on individual concerns and more on reactions to, and interactions with, the people in patients' environments.

One school of thought that aimed at addressing these limitations included a number of theorists who did not share a defining theory, but whose approaches were far different from mainstream drive and ego psychology, and they were unified by an underlying premise that human thought, emotion, and behavior reflected the influence of the social environment. These contributors are identified as the school of interpersonal psychoanalysis. (Interpersonal psychoanalysis should not be confused with interpersonal psychotherapy or IPT, developed in the 1970s as a specific style of time-limited psychotherapy focusing on interpersonal problems). Although their ideas did not have a profound overt influence on the development of psychodynamic theory, many of their notions were implicitly absorbed into the mainstream theories of object relations and self psychology which followed. The principles and philosophy of interpersonal psychoanalysis also achieved great currency with lay audiences because of their accessibility and social relevance. They will be presented here as a waystation between ego and object relations psychologies, but will not return in our examinations of affect, psychopathology, and therapy since they provided no lasting contributions to clinical practice.

HARRY STACK SULLIVAN AND THE BEGINNINGS OF INTERPERSONAL PSYCHOANALYSIS

Harry Stack Sullivan (1892–1949) was trained in the theories and techniques of Sigmund Freud and put them into practice in the treatment of severely-ill schizophrenic patients. Just as Freud had attributed meaning to the symptoms of the neuroses, Sullivan sought meaning in the psychotic content of schizophrenic thought. Unusually gifted in the art of communicating with such disturbed individuals, he was particularly impressed with their impaired capacity to relate to others. From their histories, he understood the origins of their disorders to be in reactions to their social and interpersonal environments. He took psychotic responses to be the extremes of human reaction and assumed that neurotic and normal reactions were more proximate points on the same axis.

Like Freud, Sullivan was impressed with the sexual content and primitive longings in his patients' thoughts. He fully accepted drive theory's ideas of intrapsychic conflict and repression of unconscious material. He was uneasy, however, with the theory's dogmatism and with the marginal applicability of its Victorian assumptions to his lower-class American patients. He sought to develop a theory that was more attuned to the individuality of personal experience.

Wary of filling in blank areas of knowledge with supposition, Sullivan made few attempts to imagine the content of the unconscious. By the same token, he rejected the notion of psychic structures (id, ego, and superego) and saw all mental processes as elements of energy transformation. Human motivation could be reduced to the need for satisfaction and the need for security.

Satisfaction for the infant is food, warmth, or relief of physical discomfort. Since the infant cannot provide these elements, he or she requires another person. So, the acquisition of satisfaction entails some sort of exchange between the developing individual and the environment. As the child grows, the needs for satisfaction mature to include personal contact, joy, pleasure, and emotional stimulation. More mature needs demand more sophisticated modes of interpersonal exchange. These exchanges are always imperfect at best, and the failures contribute to varying degrees of loneliness.

Security is the freedom from anxiety, but Sullivan uses anxiety in a specific and idiosyncratic fashion. For him, anxiety is an intense and potentially overwhelming fear. This fear stems not from external threats or internal conflicts. Rather, it is caught or absorbed from caretakers through "empathic linkage." The anxiety of the parent or other caretaker is conveyed to the child, and a vicious cycle ensues. While the caretaker can satisfy needs, he or she can only perpetuate anxiety, never relieve it. The developing infant can neither control nor resolve the anxiety, and it interferes with his or her ability to integrate other sources of satisfaction. As an adult, he or she retains this anxiety and passes it on as a legacy to the next generation.

The best way the child can accommodate anxiety is to discriminate between anxious and non-anxious states of experience, and identify these as "bad mother" and "good mother," respectively. (These internal identifications of states are barely, if at all, related to the actual mother of the environment.) As the child grows beyond infancy, he or she achieves the cognitive capacity to recognize that the good mother and bad mother experiences derive from the same actual person; the child also comes to appreciate that his or her own behavior can modulate the amount of anxiety in the caretaker. The acquisition of language around the first birthday is an important milestone in facilitating this capacity.

Sullivan defined the personality as "what one is" and the self as "what one takes oneself to be," i.e., a self-perception or self-representation. As the growing child assimilates more experiences that result in maternal approval, the elicitation of tenderness and the reduction of caretaker anxiety, the child, too, becomes less anxious. These non-anxious elements of personality, the experiences of security, are identified as "good-me." The areas of personality that contain anxiety in the child and evoke anxiety in the caretaker are labeled as "bad-me." Some islands of experience are connected to such intense anxiety that they are managed by amnesia for the anxiety and the events surrounding it; these elements of personality are contained in "not-me."

Eventually, the child no longer relies exclusively on the parent(s) to provide protection and limit anxiety, and the developing self tries to find a path to maximize the security of the "good-me" and avoid the anxiety of the "bad-me" and "not-me." One means to do so is the creation of fictitious others, internal representations that impose wishful characteristics on real memories of experiences with the environment. Discrepancies between these representations and real figures in the person's world are fertile ground for uncertainty and distress.

> MR. BROWN longs for the security of his father's approval. He has retained his mother's anxiety and seeks to contain it by adopting a false self-representation imitative of his father. He suffers from the contrast between his real wife and the idealized representation of his mother that he expects her to fulfill.

In this model, it is the anxiety about experiencing anxiety that is at the core of all mental disorders. Since this anxiety has interpersonal origins, the route to cure is through the interpersonal dimension as well. Health comes through reorganization of the personality to accommodate healthy interactions, and the relationship with the therapist is the crucial factor in treatment.

KAREN HORNEY AND THE INTERPERSONAL ROOTS OF NEUROSIS

Karen Horney (1885–1952), whose life was marked by considerable difficulty and disappointment in her family of origin and in her marriage, offered a view of neurosis that resembled both

Freud's and Sullivan's. Like Freud, she saw neurosis as a step on a continuum with normality. The issues and strivings of the neurotic mind are present in everyone; it is only their intensity that determines whether they become symptomatic. Like Sullivan, she was particularly attuned to the role of others in one's development and one's inner life. She saw relationships at the heart of both development and psychopathology.

Horney defined 10 *neurotic needs*, present in all but only generating distress in some:

- The need for affection and approval
- The need for a partner or someone to solve one's problems
- The need to restrict one's life and to restrain demands on others
- The need for power and control
- The need to exploit others
- The need for recognition or prestige
- The need for personal admiration and praise
- The need for personal achievement
- The need for self-sufficiency and independence
- The need for perfection

Failure to achieve any of these needs generates a degree of anxiety. In the neurotic individual, the needs are unrealistic and the anxiety intense. As the ego psychologists defined the defense mechanisms, Horney more simply clustered people's coping strategies into:

- Compliance
- Aggression
- Withdrawal

MS. GRAY retains a number of unfulfilled or incompletely fulfilled neurotic needs, including especially the needs for affection, for a partner, and for control. Her deprivation in these areas has led her to overemphasize her pursuit of exploitation of others. Her behavior manifests overt compliance with the often abusive demands of those from whom she seeks affection, while aggressive outbursts characterize her frustration with unmet needs.

Like Sullivan, Horney examined the concept of the self and its role in development and pathology. She defined the self as the core of one's being, containing his or her potential. Under optimal circumstances, if the burden of neurosis is not too great, one's self-perception is accurate and life comprises a striving toward self-realization. For the neurotic, however, perceptions are distorted and the self is split into an "ideal self," consisting of the often unattainable, and a "despised self," characterized by one's short-comings. The neurotic alternates between self-loathing and pursuit of unattainable perfection. The energy spent on this vacillation deprives the person of accurate self-perception and self-realization.

ERICH FROMM AND THE SOCIAL AND HISTORICAL CONTEXT

Coming of age in Germany during the harrowing days of World War I, Erich Fromm (1900–1980) sought explanation for the insanity of the masses. He found answers in the works of both Freud and Karl Marx and devoted his career to synthesizing the ideas of the two major figures.

Fromm's work as a psychotherapist and his experience in the world confirmed his faith in the Freudian notion of the unconscious and its substantial power. He added a premise, which was consistent with Marx's beliefs that the inner world of each individual was shaped not just by the inherited drives and the immediate family, but from the cultural and historical context into which he or she is born. The solutions people craft to the problems of the human condition lead to the establishment of social values.

Freud's patients, Fromm postulated, were burdened by the "false consciousness" of their Victorian society; it was underneath this cloak that Freud discovered their true sexual and aggressive urges. Freud's mistake, however, was to attend exclusively to the content of these urges rather than to the hypocrisy and self-deception of maintaining the social façade. The hypocrisy rather than the suppressed id, said Fromm, was the source of human distress.

 MS. WHITE has been forced by society to assume a role as wife and mother. Although she has accepted it with considerable satisfaction, she has had to submerge true ambitions of her own. With the departure of her youngest child from home and the intrusion of her newly retired husband into her domain, Ms. White comes face to face with the compromises she has had to forge over the preceding decades.

Fromm described human beings as fundamentally alone; we are at one with nature only at the moment of birth and all the rest is separation. This circumstance forces us to choose between a "productive orientation" or any of several more regressive and less adaptive orientations. The productive orientation acknowledges his or her biological and social nature, yet confronts personal choice and responsibility. The healthy life is characterized by "wanting to act as they have to act."

However, since society has not yet achieved the Marxist ideal of support for full human development, compromises are usually necessary. The other orientations (which Fromm calls "receptive," "exploitative," "hoarding," and "marketing") all entail compromises of personal choice and freedom. Each defines a particular kind of hypocrisy, and these hypocrisies underlie psychopathology.

Learning points

- The interpersonal theorists opened the door to the examination of the role of other persons in human development and psychopathology.
- Harry Stack Sullivan clarified the role of the social environment in the formation of the human mind and personality. He painted a lifelong human struggle between the need for satisfaction and the need for security.
- Karen Horney saw human relationships as the core element of development and mental life. She identified a number of neurotic needs and the coping strategies that people mobilize to deal with the frustration of those needs.
- Erich Fromm emphasized the social and historical context of individual psychology. He paid particular tension to the role of hypocrisy, resulting from trying to fit into one's social environment, in the genesis of psychopathology.

RECOMMENDED READINGS

Boeree CG. *Erich Fromm.* http://www.ship.edu/;cboeree/fromm.html, 1997.

Mitchell SA, Black MJ. *Freud and Beyond: A History of Modern Psychoanalytic Thought.* New York: Basic Books, 1995.

Sullivan HS. *The Interpersonal Theory of Psychiatry.* New York: Norton, 1953.

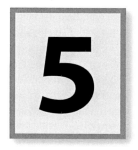

Object Relations Theory

"Very few people love others for what they are; rather, they love what they lend them, their own selves, their own idea of them."
—Johann Wolfgang von Goethe

LEARNING OBJECTIVES

The reader will be able to:

1. List the principles common to all object relations theories.
2. Define the major theorists' views of human motivation and drives.
3. Define the major theorists' views of the nature and origin of the ego, id, and superego.

Sigmund Freud's drive psychology, like any revolutionary theory, raised as many issues as it explained. Perhaps its biggest shortcoming was that it remained a one-organism psychology. The "objects" in Freud's world were essentially interchangeable. If the parent did not overly neglect or traumatize the infant, he or she would mature according to plan. And since the clinical practice driven by the theory dealt with such disorders as compulsions, phobias, and hysterical conversions, the explanations were mostly sufficient.

The ego psychologists added texture to the model by describing in more detail the intricacies of the structure ego and the

73

elements of development. They succeeded in beginning to build a general psychology that could explain normal as well as pathological development. In doing so, they accomplished two things. First, they were forced to look more carefully at the particular interpersonal environments of patients and normal children, and discovered that caregivers and others were not faceless, but made specific contributions. Second, because of the clinical success of their theories, they brought patients with problems not reducible to Oedipal conflicts into psychoanalysis and began to glimpse the pre-Oedipal nature of some psychopathology and the interpersonal sources of much psychic distress. These developments forced theorists to think more precisely about the role of others in the development of the human mind and in the genesis of psychopathology.

The thinkers of the interpersonal school made forays in these directions, but none attracted the critical mass of followers to develop any momentum. Such a nucleus did emerge (primarily in Great Britain) in the 1920s and 1930s and gained both traction and persistence as the object relations school of psychoanalytic theory. Because they were reworking many Freudian ideas, they had to retain his vocabulary and a nominal loyalty to drive theory. Each created his or her own language and focused on the specifics of his or her ideas that differentiated them from the rest. Thus we know these theorists today mostly by their disparities. It is important first to emphasize what is held in common by the object relations theorists before specifying their distinctions.

At its core, each theory maintains that people develop by interacting with real people in their environments, and they develop internal worlds that contain representations of these experiences. These representations shape how infants and children develop, and they shape how adults anticipate and perceive the interpersonal events in their worlds. The nature of these relationships profoundly affects the structures of id, ego, and superego. These experiences are recreated in the transference situation, where they can be analyzed and altered. (See Table 5-1.)

The differences among the object relations theories include:

- The extent to which they differ with Freud's drive/structure model
- Their definitions of critical developmental issues and events
- Their views of human motivation

TABLE 5-1	*Principles Common to Object Relations Theories*

- Early interactions between infant and caretaker are the foundation of attitudes toward the self and others. The infant develops characteristic interactional patterns and a repertoire of defenses and strengths.

- Problems with early object relations produce troubled adult relationships and a wide range of maladaptive personality characteristics. These early problems typically include early object loss as well as experiences with caretakers who are neglectful, intrusive, unempathic, and/or abusive.

- Clinical patients bring their characteristic patterns of interaction into therapy, where they are predictably activated in the transference.

- Therapeutic change in individuals with disturbed object relations results from reparative experiences within the psychotherapy as well as clarifying interpretations.

The theorists who best represent the different approaches to these differences are Melanie Klein, Margaret Mahler, W.R.D. Fairbairn, Donald Winnicott, and Otto Kernberg.

MELANIE KLEIN: AGGRESSION AND "PHANTASY"

From an epistemological perspective, Melanie Klein (1882–1960) offered a distinct contribution to psychoanalysis. Untrained as a scientist or philosopher, she drew conclusions based not on the recollections of neurotic adults, but on direct observations of children at play and in analysis. Since children could not give words to the abstractions underlying their behavior, she was forced to speculate about their meaning. The theories she devised, rich in imagery and passion, added new depth particularly to considerations of fantasy and aggression. Study of Klein is complicated by the evolution of her ideas over time. For our purposes, we will outline the latest versions of her theories, together with those elements of earlier versions that were never rescinded.

For Sigmund Freud, drives existed by themselves; the entities to which they attached themselves became objects by definition. Klein could not accept this model and held that drives are inherently object-directed. Even an infant cannot experience libido without a libidinal object. She soon came to find aggression to be a more influential force than libido in childhood development. Both aggression and libido, in her view, are bound to specific objects. Further, emotions are not neurotic manifestations of drive impulses, they are inherent features of the drives themselves: libido is loving; aggression is hateful.

Aggression for Klein was manifest in the child's dominant aim to possess and control, and to ultimately destroy the objects in his or her environment. Where Freud had formulated the Oedipal conflict as one of libidinal desire for a prohibited object, Klein saw it as a struggle for power, possession, and destruction. As in the Freudian version, a result of the struggle is the fear of retaliation. For Freud, it was jealous reprisal for possession of the mother; for Klein, angry retribution by the assaulted father. Even further, because Klein saw object-directed aggression at work from birth on, she postulated the existence of a primitive Oedipal complex even in infancy.

Klein's most substantial contribution may have been her new formulation of fantasy. In drive psychology, fantasy was an adaptive substitute for something undesirable in the real environment. In ego psychology, it was a modality for organizing perceptions. Klein instead viewed it as the singular substrate of all mental processes. She defined an inborn, unconscious function, whose content and images are phylogenetically inherited. Fantasy could be seen as the mental representation of drive instinct. Fantasy, Klein maintained, was primary, and the infant was born with a densely populated object world. Perceptions of real persons were distorted to fit the templates of this inner world.

Klein outlined the stages of development into what she called "positions," defining constellations of phantasy and emotion.

- The *paranoid position* (later called the *paranoid-schizoid* position) occupies the first 3 months of life. The infant organizes phantasies and experiences into good and bad objects. The homogeneity of these objects leaves the child vulnerable to abandonment or destruction, hence the paranoia.

- By the second quarter of the first year, the child enters the *depressive* position. Klein posits that the child at this stage begins to realize that the good and bad mother are the same person, but still believes in the destructive power of his or her own aggressive impulses. As a result, the child is fearful of the effects of his or her hostile wishes on the object of libidinal attachment.

> MS. GRAY directed aggressive impulses toward her mother for failing to resist and deflect her father's cruelty. Worried that this aggression hurt her mother and the internalized representation of her mother, she is left with a predisposition to depressed feelings. Unable to tolerate the internal consequences of this hostility, she directs it at multiple external objects, which play symbolic roles in her phantasy world.

The depressive position is never fully resolved, and psychological life is a continuing pursuit of reparation for the harm done. The entire Oedipal complex is now a vehicle for undoing the effects of depressive anxiety. In less fortunate individuals, the picture is even more complicated as unresolved remnants of the paranoid position restrict the available range of mental operations.

Since Klein's link between drives and objects was so fundamental, it required a reformulation of the mental structures that housed them. Ego was no longer a developmental outgrowth of the conflict between aggression and libido within the id. Instead, ego was a medium for love and connection; id, for hate and destruction. Both, therefore, had to be present from birth. For Freud, the central conflict was between drive and reality. For Klein it was a war between love and hate.

MARGARET MAHLER: SEPARATION AND INDIVIDUATION

Margaret Mahler (1897–1985) was a pediatrician before becoming a psychoanalyst. Like Klein, she formed her hypotheses with direct observations of children. Her work addressed the question of the sources of human individuality. She was attracted to Hartmann's notions of adaptation and extended them to describe adaptation to the interpersonal, human environment.

Mahler outlined phases of human psychological development:

- *Normal autism,* occupying just the first few weeks of life, is focused on satisfying needs and reducing discomfort or tension. The infant uses hallucinations to gratify his or her wishes until they are fulfilled in actuality; reality testing is nonexistent.

■ The *normal symbiotic phase* lasts from about the ages of 4 weeks to 4 months. The developing body becomes more aware of external stimuli. The infant is aware of the mother, but identifies her as a single unit with himself or herself. Experiences are classified as either good or bad, and memory traces begin to get laid down consistent with those divisions.

■ *Separation-individuation* characterizes the remainder of human psychological development. Separation is the emergence of the child from symbiotic unity; individuation is the acquisition of personal characteristics. This large phase is divided into 4 subphases:

  ● *Differentiation*—From ages 5 to 10 months, the child perceives himself or herself as distinct from mother and eventually separates mother from others.

  ● *Practicing*—From about 10 to 18 months of age, the child, who can now crawl and explore, expands his or her sphere of interest. Mahler specifically identifies upright locomotion as the marker of the "psychological birth" of the child. While in love with the world around, the child frequently returns to mother as home base.

  ● *Rapprochement*—From 18 to about 30 months of age, the child begins to realize that mother is a truly separate person. The development of language helps the child bridge this potentially frightening gap. As reality testing improves, infantile grandiosity wanes, but frustration rises. As the child alternates between intense need for mother and hostile rejection of her, splitting becomes the primary adaptive mechanism.

  ● *Libidinal object constancy*—The rest of life entails the merging of split object representations. The child, and later the adult, learns that persons in the environment remain constant even as experiences with them vary from good to bad.

Like Hartmann, Mahler conceived of an originally undifferentiated matrix of id and ego components. For Hartmann, the need to survive in the physical world drove the evolution of the ego. For Mahler, objects constituted anything that had contact with the child. Objects were not tied to drives. The symbiotic investment in the object, particularly the mother, gave rise to the evolution of libido out of a previously undifferentiated matrix of drive energy. Hostility directed at objects outside the symbiotic circle gave rise to the differentiation of aggression. Ego arose when the child was able to await and expect satisfaction, which originally could come only from others, i.e., with the beginning of the capacity for memory.

The origin of the ego and the differentiation of libido, from their respective undifferentiated matrices, thus requires a reliable other. If the hungry infant is not fed or if the crying infant is not soothed, there is no positive object experience to serve as the core of libido; no positive memory traces can be established to serve as foundation for ego. Mahler referred to the "ordinarily devoted mother" who could fulfill these criteria, and more generally to the "average expectable environment" which was necessary for normal development.

MR. BROWN successfully separated from mother. In the process of individuation, he experienced her as somewhat inadequate by virtue of her passivity. The tense and unemotional family environment failed to provide a sufficient anchor for his developing libidinal attachments. His repetitive adult behavior mirrors the child's need for rapprochement. He retains a high degree of dependency on external objects for validation, and he struggles for libidinal object constancy.

W.R.D. FAIRBAIRN:
OBJECT-SEEKING AND MOTIVATION

W.R.D. (Ronald) Fairbairn (1889–1964), working in relative isolation in Scotland, had more influence posthumously than he did in life on the British School of object relations. From the beginning, he doubted the drive theory of motivation. To his observation, libido is object-seeking, not pleasure-seeking. The pursuit of pleasure and sexual gratification is only a vehicle for connection to others. He saw no need for a structure id, but considered the ego to be the container of psychic energies; it is a set of organizing and mediating functions, all in pursuit of object relations. Where aggression exists, it is a reaction to libidinal frustration, not an impulse of its own.

From these principles it follows that development is not a matter of structure-building as it was for the drive and ego psychologists, but an evolution in modes of relating.

- *Infantile dependence* is characterized by the child's sense of merger with mother. The world and the self are a single object. The infant's survival depends on mother's presence and attunement.
- The *transitional stage* constitutes a long process of separation. Relationships emerge based on differentiation and exchange. Relinquishing the merger of infantile dependence, the child fears the loss of objects.
- *Mature dependence* features a healthy, mutual interdependence between adults. The selfishness of infantile dependence and the barter of the transitional phase give way to the altruistic generosity of adulthood. Of course, the transition is never complete, and the insecurities of the transitional phase are present throughout life.

 MS. WHITE successfully traversed the early stages of development. Now she struggles to achieve the ideal of mature dependence. On the one hand, what seemed like altruistic devotion to motherhood when her children were at home now feels more like hurtful over-involvement. The altered marital boundaries since her husband's retirement challenge her to define the extent of her dependency on him.

The natural, or primary, objects of the ego are other people. But reality interferes with the mother–infant bond and requires the creation of internal objects. To contain the bad or frustrating objects, the ego splits. The *central ego* consists of positive objects and experiences; it constitutes the conscious, relational aspects of ego function. The exciting, provocative image of mother, intensely attractive, is split into an exciting object, which is contained in the *libidinal ego*. The unavailable mother gives rise to a frustrating object representation, contained in the *anti-libidinal ego*. If object relations remain unsatisfactory, the splits persist; otherwise (and normally) they merge into a healthy ego and object world.

Psychopathology, for Fairbairn, reflected the basic struggle between intense longings for contact and the irreconcilable features of others in external reality. If the ego is forced to remain fragmented to maintain contact with the split representations of others, a genuine self cannot emerge. (See Chapter 6.)

Thus, therapy must be aimed at unifying the split elements of ego. The patient, despite his or her fear of being retraumatized, must come to experience the therapist as a good object. With a strong, real, and transferential relationship, the therapist helps the patient surrender bad objects from repression, loosen the libidinal ties to them, and reattach them into an integrated, genuine adult self. (See Chapter 8.)

D.W. WINNICOTT: THE TRUE AND FALSE SELVES

Donald W. Winnicott (1896–1971), like Margaret Mahler, was originally a pediatrician. Even though he practiced psychoanalysis with psychotic adults, he rejected Freud's view of the depravity of mankind. Instead, he saw human nature as basically good. From his observations of children and their mothers, he emphasized the role of the specific interpersonal environment in shaping that nature for better or worse. A substantial number of his phrases and the ideas connected to children and their mothers have become part of the permanent psychological vocabulary.

"There is no such thing as a baby without a mother," he declared. There exists instead a nursing couple, bonded more by emotion than by the physical tie of Mahler's stage of symbiosis. Proper development requires *good enough mothering*, which entails the beginning a stage of *primary maternal preoccupation* and lasting 2 to 3 weeks. For the first few months of life, the mother is intensely attuned to the child's desires. She provides a *holding environment* in which the child is protected from discomfort. Further, she anticipates the baby's needs as the infant is on the verge of summoning them up in fantasy. She also provides a mirror for the baby, confirming his or her existence; and a nondemanding presence during times of rest so the child can simply exist, allowing spontaneous gestures to emerge to which the mother can respond. Briefly, Winnicott describes a requirement for perfect mothering, with flawless and constant attunement to the infant's unspoken wishes. Once the mother has fostered this illusion of omnipotence, her inevitable failures can allow the infant to learn about reality.

The developing child soon evolves needs for object relationships separate from early drive needs. The maternal position, her
attitudes, and emotions, become more important than the
content of her gratifications. Such object relations become struc-
turalized into the self. If the mother does not protect the
omnipotent illusion, or if she intrudes on the formless, quiet
periods with needs of her own, the child develops a *false self*,
compliant and adaptive to the parental needs and expectations.
Because the baby is still dependent on its mother for survival, the
true self must be buried.

MR. BROWN lacked the "good enough mothering" that would have
allowed him to consolidate his true self. His preoccupied and distracted
parents were insufficiently attuned to foster his sense of omnipotence
and guide him through its expectable frustrations. In an attempt at
repair, he imitates his father; but this imitation represents a pursuit of a
false self. The conflict between true and false selves is manifest in his
social timidity and his professional pattern of self-defeat.

In growing from infantile omnipotence to an adaptive relationship with the external world, the child makes use of language and motor functions. Importantly, he or she also relies on
a *transitional object*. This object (often something like a blanket or
teddy bear) occupies a vague space between illusion and reality.
The infant imagines a breast he or she can create out of wishing
alone; the toddler knows he or she has to ask for things that
may or may not be forthcoming. The transitional object sits
between these stages. It is not entirely illusory and it does not
belong completely to the cold, external world. Neither the child
nor the parent questions its source or its nature. Adults outside
the intimate circle of parent and child regard the attachment as
cute, though irrational. Significantly, since the transitional
object is the first creation of the child's mind, it may be seen as
the beginning of human creativity.

While Winnicott professed allegiance to Freud's model, he rel-
egates the drives to a marginal position compared with the need
for connection; and he has little use for the structures of id and ego.
Aggression is not a primary drive but a direct result of frustration
of libidinal wishes. A failure of good enough mothering prevents
the emergence of the true self, and most psychopathology repre-

sents a stage of developmental arrest at the point where proper parenting would have facilitated the emergence of the true self, or at the stage where parental needs forced the naissance of elements of the false self. (See Chapter 7.)

Psychoanalytic cure for Winnicott required the direct provision of missing developmental needs. In the holding environment of the therapy, the patient would experience the freedom to make contact with his or her true self and rid himself or herself of the fixations of the false self. (See Chapter 9.)

OTTO KERNBERG: THE BORDERLINE MIND

Otto Kernberg (1928–) emerged in the late 20th century as the leading spokesperson for object relations theory. Using the language of the drive model, he presented the conclusions he drew from extensive work with patients with borderline and narcissistic personalities. His theories emphasize the centrality of affect and the profound importance of splitting, in development and experience.

Kernberg's system is built on the *basic relational unit*: the image of the object, the image of the self, *and* the affect in play (derived from the drive which is active at the time). The infant, the toddler, and the child progress through multiple such experiences in the process of forming psychic structures and personality:

- Early on, the infant internalizes these experiences by *introjection*, in which self and object are hardly differentiated and the affect is a violent and unmodified drive derivative.
- Later, introjection is replaced by *identification*, in which the child is able to appreciate the separate roles played by self and object, and affect is somewhat modulated.
- *Ego identity*, the most mature form of internalization, organizes the particular elements of self and object under the synthetic functions of the fully formed ego; affect is well modulated.

In the earliest stages of existence, drive energy is undifferentiated and physiologically determined. In the course of accumulating relational experiences, the affective coloration of each basic relational unit, love or hate, identifies it as good or bad. The objects within each unit become invested with drive energy, which then sorts itself into libido and aggression, depending on the affective context of the associated experiences. Hate exists before aggression; love, before libido. The drives serve as organizers of the internalized relational units.

 MS. GRAY'S early relational experiences were colored by extremely negative affects of fear and sadness, more of hate than of love. These experiences were organized into a deep reservoir of aggressive drive energy. The aggression is so intense, and the experiences of love have been so rare, that she has remained unable to merge her adult perception of others beyond this primitive splitting. The lack of modulation has blocked the formation of an effective adult ego, preventing the perception of others in her environment as constant figures. Instead she perceives people according to the affective tone of the moment.

In infancy, there are originally no psychic structures. Perception is a function of a forerunner of the ego. Ego is born as a product of introjection of object experiences. As ego introjects multiple pleasant and unpleasant images, desirable and frightening emotions, it must repress those which are too upsetting to maintain in awareness. This repository becomes the id. Superego is a later differentiation, providing the locus of hostile, punitive images as well as lofty ego ideals. Eventually, splitting becomes an untenable process and the ego progresses to ambivalence, holding simultaneous good and bad properties of an object in a single representation. (See Figure 5-1.)

Although Kernberg's model uses Freud's terms and superficially espouses loyalties to the drive model, it in fact turns drive theory upside down. For Kernberg, object relations are primary; they exist before any of the structures. Affects flow directly from the nature of the object experiences and are managed primarily by splitting. These experiences actually create the drives. Since affect and splitting are ego functions, the ego creates the id out of repressed drive derivatives. This model, though complicated and cumbersome, offers more complete explanations of pre-Oedipal function and severe adult pathology than any prior system. It represents the apotheosis of the evolution of object relations theories in its replacement of nearly all principles of drive psychology.

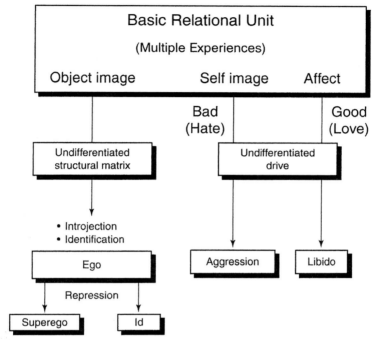

FIGURE 5-1 ▦ Kernberg's Model of Drive and Structure.

REFINEMENT OF THE THEORIES

The evolution of ego psychology made it necessary for theorists to direct their attention to the world surrounding the developing and functioning individual. The object relations theorists jumped to this task. Sharing the principles of the role of others in shaping the person, they derived different schemes of drive and structure, ranging from the modest modifications of Klein and Mahler to the near-complete rejection of the drive-structure model by Winnicott and Kernberg. (See Table 5-2.) These diverse views persist without much accommodation. The increasing complexity and idiosyncrasies required to support the object relations theories made them inaccessible to many practitioners and epistemologically undesirable to many theorists. These considerations contributed to the alternative, or parallel, development of the school of self psychology.

TABLE 5-2 | Comparison of Major Object Relations Theories

Theorist	Origin and Role of Drives	Origin and Role of Structures	Major Developmental Themes
Melanie Klein	Aggressive and libidinal drives are inborn. They are separate from birth. Drives are inherently object-directed. Aggression is much more powerful and important than libido.	Id and ego are present in nearly mature states from birth. They serve to meet the demands of the drives.	Conflict between love and hate is central to all development. Phantasies are inborn and evolve to contain images of objects and to manage the conflict of love and hate.
Margaret Mahler	Drives originate in an undifferentiated matrix. Symbiotic investment in objects gives rise to libido. Hostility to objects outside the symbiotic sphere differentiates into aggression.	Structures originate in an undifferentiated matrix. Ego results from maturation of memory and the ability to obtain gratification from objects. Id is what is left behind.	Separation and individuation follow a predictable pattern. Development relies on the availability of dependable objects.
W.R.D. Fairbairn	There are no drives in the traditional sense. The child naturally strives for libidinal connection. Aggressive urges arise when this aim is frustrated.	There is no id, only ego. The frustration of impulses toward connection leads to splits in the ego.	Modes of relating to objects become more complex and mature. Development of drives and structures is irrelevant.
D.W. Winnicott	Libido is primary and is present from birth. The frustration of libido directs some of its energy into the creation of the aggressive drive.	Relations with objects yield the formation of a true self and a false self. Id and ego are irrelevant.	Object relations become independent aims of development, separate from drive-based needs. The reconciliation of true and false selves defines the individual.
Otto Kernberg	The child is born with unmodified and undifferentiated drive energy. Experience with objects, colored by affective context, separates aggression from libido.	Affects and perception exist before structures. Experiences with objects are organized by introjection and identification into the structure ego. Unacceptable elements of experience are split and repressed into the structure id.	Affects are organized by relational experiences. Primitive splitting is replaced by more adaptive modes of containing hate and obtaining love.

Learning points

- All object relations theories describe an internal object world that results from early experience with others in the environment.
- Melanie Klein emphasized the role of aggression and phylogenetically inherited "phantasy" in shaping the object world.
- Margaret Mahler described the process by which the child separates from mother and becomes an individual.
- W.R.D. Fairbairn emphasized that drives are inherently object-seeking.
- D.W. Winnicott introduced the concepts of "good enough mothering," the "holding environment," and the "transitional object."
- Otto Kernberg emphasized the roles of affect and splitting in the origins of drive and structure.

RECOMMENDED READINGS

Greenberg JR, Mitchell SA. *Object Relations in Psychoanalytic Theory.* Cambridge: Harvard University Press, 1983.

Kernberg OF. Psychoanalytic object relations theories. In: BE Moore, BD Fine. *Psychoanalysis: The Major Concepts.* New Haven, CT: Yale University Press, 1995:450–462.

Mishne JM. *The Evolution and Application of Clinical Theory.* New York, NY: Free Press, 1993.

Scharff JS, Scharff DE. *Object Relations Individual Therapy.* Northvale, NJ: Jason Aronson Inc., 1998.

Self Psychology

"Self-love, my liege, is not so vile a sin as self-neglecting."
—*William Shakespeare*

LEARNING OBJECTIVES

The reader will be able to:

1. Define self and selfobject from the perspective of self psychology.
2. Describe the bipolar self.
3. Outline the process of development from the self psychological perspective.

Ego psychology had enriched and broadened the arena of psychodynamic thought, but left two problems. First, it was a one-person psychology, treating the mind of the individual as a self-contained entity. Second, as its successes accumulated, people availed themselves of analysis whose problems were more deep-rooted than the Oedipal-level conflicts addressed by drive and ego theories. Object relations theories addressed both of these issues, finding principles to describe the interpersonal dimensions of the psyche and concurrently addressing pre-Oedipal development and serious personality pathology. A very different approach to the same problems arose in the United States in the 1960s.

Heinz Kohut (1913–1981) came to Chicago from Vienna. He rapidly achieved prominence in the prevailing school of ego psychology and was widely anticipated to become Heinz Hartmann's successor. But his clinical experience brought home the shortcomings of ego psychology. He did not find object relations theory to be a satisfying answer because it was so abstract, seemingly too distant from human experience to be of scientific verifiability or clinical utility. He reformulated the theories of the mind in a radical fashion as self psychology. Its critical elements are the normality of narcissism, the centrality of selfobject experiences, and the role of empathy in development, investigation, and treatment.

THE SELF AND SELFOBJECTS

Self psychology rejects the notions of drive and structure as artificial constructs divorced from experience. Kohut saw them as simply unnecessary for a description of the mind. The only structure for which he saw a purpose was the self. Freud had not differentiated between self and ego. (He used the German word for self, *das Ich*, to name what was subsequently translated as "ego.") Hartmann, describing the ego in greater detail, defined the self as the representation of the whole person within the structure ego. Object relations theorists mostly considered the self similarly to be a representation of a special kind of object within the ego, parallel to the representations of external objects.

Eliminating the ego, self psychology defines the self as the central agency of identity and individuality, the constant thread of unique personhood that binds life's experiences. Metaphorically, it is considered a structure because it is continuous and changes only very slowly. It is a "supraordinate" construct that comprises the entire range of experience over time. But the self cannot be directly observed or experienced and is known only by the manifestations to which it gives rise: features of self-esteem and of distress.

Kohut's observations, like those of the object relations theorists, led him to conclude that the self cannot exist in isolation. He posited a self that accumulates experiences of interaction with others in the environment. These interactions shared between self and other are *selfobject experiences*, usually known less clumsily as *selfobjects*. Note that the selfobject of self psychology is not an external person, a structure of its own, or even an internal representation of another (as in object relations theory). Rather it is an experience necessary for the nurture and/or maintenance of the self.

The need for selfobjects is a lifelong one. There is no self without selfobjects, and this dynamic network of experience is called the *selfobject matrix*. Much as Winnicott had rejected the need for the structure ego and proceeded to describe the evolution of energy of the self in a world of objects, Kohut elucidated the evolution of the self within the selfobject matrix.

THE BIPOLAR SELF

If the self is the center, or the entirety, of mental life, then narcissism can no longer be seen as a transitional phase or as a pathological residue in adult life. Recognizing narcissism as a lifelong focus, self psychology defines the needs of the developing self that foster healthy narcissism and the balances that must be struck to avoid pathological manifestations of narcissistic development. Giving a framework to what he heard from patients, Kohut postulated the existence of the *bipolar self*. The two poles of the self-object matrix that define the development and maintenance of the self are the pole of self-assertive ambitions and the pole of values and ideals. (See Figure 6-1.)

The presence of a *mirroring selfobject* (a parent or other vital figure who reflects positively the qualities, capacities, and accomplishments of the self) fosters the emergence of the *grandiose self*. At the same time, the presence of an *idealizable selfobject* (a person, figure, or function that provides goals and aims for the developing self) fosters the emergence of an internalized figure of ideals and aspirations, the *idealized parental imago*. The two poles sing a duet: "I am good" and "I can be great."

MS. GRAY was raised in an environment deficient in both mirroring and idealizable selfobjects. As a result, she lacks the capacities for regulating either affect or self-esteem. Contemporary experiences buffet her mercilessly, and she engages in continuing and repeated efforts to find the missing infantile selfobject experiences in her adult life.

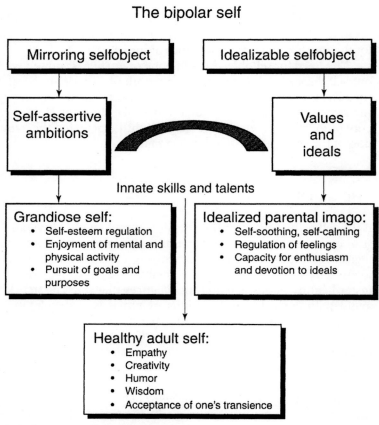

The bipolar self

FIGURE 6-1 ▩ The bipolar self.

Note that, in self psychology, grandiosity is not inherently pathological. To the contrary, it is, in proper form, necessary for healthy self-development. The presence of idealized targets implies that the self is not perfect, creating a "tension arc" between the two poles. This tension functions creatively under desirable circumstances to foster the emergence and refinement of innate skills and talents.

Appropriate development of the grandiose self brings about the capacity to regulate self-esteem and to enjoy mental and physical activity. Development of the idealized pole yields the capacity to soothe oneself under stress, to regulate emotions, to devote oneself to ideals, and to experience enthusiasm. From the innate skills and talents of the nuclear self emerge the essence of what Kohut defined as the features of the healthy adult self:

- Empathy
- Creativity
- Humor
- Wisdom
- Acceptance of one's own transience

MS. WHITE, having received sufficient mirroring from idealizable parents, displays in middle age the qualities of wisdom and creativity. Her ability to mobilize humor is strained by her current circumstances. Generally able to be empathic, her self-absorption at present makes it difficult for her to do so with both her husband and her son. She is having considerable trouble accepting her own transience.

EMPATHY

Central to this entire scheme is the concept of *empathy*. In self psychology, the term has commonly been defined as "vicarious introspection," "temporary indwelling," and "experience-near observation." It is the process of seeing another's world through his or her eyes and knowing what the other is feeling.

The specific term "empathy" is used within this theory to describe a number of functions:

- At the most abstract level, empathy defines the field of psychoanalysis. As an epistemologist, Kohut maintained that any science is defined by the object of its study and the method by which data is obtained. In the physical sciences, the objects are external and concrete, therefore the methods are observational. In psychoanalysis, the field of study is the inner workings of the mind, which are not accessible with the instruments or methods of the physical sciences. The field of observation is defined by the analyst's investigation of the subjective experience of the analysand through transiently placing himself or herself inside the subject's experience.

▤ Similarly, then, empathy is the tool for acquiring data. It is the means by which the psychotherapist enters into the world of the patient without losing his or her own identity and objectivity. Empathic observation is supraordinate to noting facial expression or the explicit content of the patient's speech or what most other people might experience in the patient's situation.

▤ At the most functional level, empathy serves a sustaining function. In the therapeutic setting, it provides implicit affirmation and mirroring. The knowledge that the therapist can perceive and comprehend the patient's experience makes it feel valid.

Although empathy is thus defined primarily in the context of therapy, it serves an irreplaceable function in normal development. In order to provide selfobject needs, the other person must have some empathic sense of what those needs are. The ideal empathic mother is in tune with her child closely enough that she can sense the source of the infant's distress early and specifically and will respond to it without delay. A mother who waits for her infant to cry before responding, who experiments with feeding, changing diapers, and cuddling because she cannot guess the source of the child's distress, fails to provide such empathic sustenance. While purists of both the object relations and self psychology schools reject the comparison, the similarity of Kohut's ideally empathic selfobject and Winnicott's "good enough mother" are striking.

DEVELOPMENT, COHESION, AND FRAGMENTATION

Kohut recognized, however, that no mother, no selfobject of any sort, can always be perfectly in tune. Every selfobject function is vulnerable to the occasional—and inevitable—failure of empathy. In an environment marked by a preponderance of empathic attunement, such failures constitute *optimal frustration* and force the developing self to absorb selfobject functions into the self, a process called *transmuting internalization*. This process does not create new abilities de novo but facilitates the maturation and expression of inherent potential in the self.

As the child grows, the nature of selfobject needs changes. In the age of the Freudian Oedipal period, the child needs nonseductive confirmation of his or her sexual identity by the parent of the opposite sex and nonaggressive acceptance of his or her competetive strivings by the parent of the same sex. In the latency years, the child needs selfobjects as models for imitation outside the family circle; he or she often uses teachers and sports figures for this purpose. The adolescent, coming to recognize his or her parents' inevitable shortcomings, de-idealizes these early selfobjects and turns to peers for more mature versions of these functions. In adulthood, marriage and parenthood bring the challenges of obtaining selfobject satisfaction from spouses and children without using them destructively. In middle age, people typically turn to more abstract and transcendent sources of selfobject fulfillment such as art and spirituality. In late life, the task of acceptance of one's mortality comes to the fore and selfobject needs are focused on equanimity and acceptance.

If all the ingredients are present and their integration is successful, the result is a *cohesive* self, i.e., a self with a sense of constancy and internal reliability. At the opposite pole from self-cohesion is *self-fragmentation*, a sense of emptiness, a feeling that one's self-experiences do not fit together.

Cohesion and fragmentation form a continuum of states. Any individual possesses some degree of cohesion, but it is never complete. The terms also describe transient states of the self. That is, a generally cohesive self, under severe stress, may fragment, as in a situation of extreme psychic trauma. Less obviously, a generally fragmented self can cohere transiently, as when an individual with a serious personality disorder is able to manage an emergency successfully because there is no other option.

As will be described in Chapter 7, all psychopathology is seen as products of the fragmentation of the self. A chronically fragmented self is manifest in one of the disorders of personality. A cohesive self that fragments under strain exhibits any of the range of specific psychopathological symptoms and syndromes previously characterized as neuroses. The therapy of these disorders, by necessity, consists of providing empathic attunement, paying attention to the inevitable moments of optimal frustration, interpreting the selfobject needs, and thereby enhancing the cohesiveness of the self.

Learning points

■ Heinz Kohut rejected the drives and the structures of the earlier psychologies and described in detail the single structure of the self.

■ Between the self's two poles of grandiosity and idealization lies a tension arc of innate talents and capacities.

■ The self has a lifelong need for selfobject experiences that contribute to a sense of permanence, identity, reliability, and self-esteem.

■ Psychopathology is the manifestation of fragmentation of the self, either chronically in personality disorders or transiently in symptoms and syndromes.

RECOMMENDED READINGS

Martin JI. Self psychology theory. In: Lehmann P, Cody N. *Theoretical Perspectives for Direct Social Work Practice*. New York: Springer Publishing Co., 2001.

Ornstein PH, Kay J. Development of psychoanalytic self psychology: a historical-conceptual overview. In: Tasman A, Goldfinger SM, Kaufman CA, eds. *American Psychiatric Press Review of Psychiatry*. Vol. 9. Washington, D.C.: American Psychiatric Press, 1990:299–322.

Siegel AM. *Heinz Kohut and the Psychology of the Self*. London: Routledge, 1996.

Wolf ES. *Treating the Self: Elements of Clinical Self Psychology*. New York: Guilford Press, 1988.

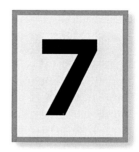

Affect and Psychopathology

"What a battle a man must fight everywhere to maintain his standing army of thoughts, and march with them in orderly array through the always hostile country! How many enemies there are to sane thinking! Every soldier has succumbed to them before he enlists for those other battles."

—Henry David Thoreau

LEARNING OBJECTIVES

The reader will be able to:

1. Describe the drive theories of anxiety and psychopathology.
2. Describe the ego psychological theories of emotional and behavioral pathology.
3. Describe the object relations theories of affective disorders and psychopathology.
4. Describe the self psychological approach to affective and behavioral disturbances.

THEORY, AFFECT, AND PSYCHOPATHOLOGY

The preceding chapters have outlined the major philosophies of the structures and functions of the mind and their normal development. Each scheme describes a complicated system with multiple opportunities for processes to go awry. Since the major

97

psychologies were derived from clinical practice, and since clinicians only become involved when things go wrong, each school of thought takes its own approach to the genesis and nature of psychopathology. Each school's view of normal development and function is intimately linked to its view of how things go amiss.

Moods, of course, are a vital part of normal mental life. Emotions color our individual worlds and add a special dimension to experience. In clinical practice, however, and in the theories that underlie it, emotions are considered a special case of psychopathology, stemming from the same roots as disorders of thought, perception, and behavior. (Perhaps it is for this reason that most of the literature uses the term "affect" to describe what is more precisely identified as "mood," or, in everyday language, "emotion.") Therefore our review of psychopathology will incorporate each theory's view of emotional states.

DRIVE PSYCHOLOGY

The original topographic model of drive psychology generated a schema of psychopathology that was as mechanical as the underlying theory itself and was of severely limited clinical applicability. From about 1885 to 1897, the focus was on the so-called "actual neuroses," namely neurasthenia and anxiety neuroses. In certain individuals who had been rendered neuropathic by congenital or hereditary predisposition, unhygienic sexual practices produced symptoms directly. Excessive masturbation or nocturnal emissions yielded neurasthenia, a condition marked by lassitude, fatigue, and somatic symptoms such as headache and dyspepsia. Sexual frustration or sexual activity that did not result in gratification produced anxiety neuroses, marked by persistent anxiety punctuated by anxiety attacks.

This model of "dammed-up libido" lacked enough explanatory capacity to survive without substantial modification. As psychoanalysts became more attentive to the nature and workings of the drives, a second model emerged and held sway from about 1897 to 1923. Energy was the domain of the drives, not of the affect itself. Emotions were now considered to be drive derivatives, and psychopathology was the result of conflicts originating from the drives. The classical formulation of hysteria formed the bedrock of psychoanalytic explanation of behavioral pathology.

Freud and Josef Breuer examined and treated a number of patients with "hysteria," i.e., symptoms of muscular or sensory impairment not traceable to any somatic cause. Drawing on the work of Jean Martin Charcot and Pierre Janet in Paris, they at first hypnotized their hysterical patients and discovered emotional conflicts that were being symbolically represented in the hysterical symptoms. For example, in the case of "Fraulein Elizabeth von R.," the patient's younger sister became sick during her pregnancy. Fraulein von R. went for a walk with her sister's husband. Returning home a few days later, she awoke with unexplained pain and weakness in her legs. Under hypnosis, it became evident that she desired her brother-in-law but of course could not acknowledge this forbidden attraction. In the topographic model of the time, her desire was suppressed, and her guilt was manifest as pain and weakness in the very legs that took her on the walk. Hypnosis soon proved unnecessary as Freud and Breuer found patients could recall "forgotten" events when fully awake, and the other cases they studied supported the same formula:

> An unacceptable emotion stems from the drives. It cannot be experienced in the system Cs (conscious), so it is relegated to the system UCs (unconscious). Since there is no avenue for direct resolution of the conflicted emotional state, the energy deriving from the drive is manifest in physical symptoms, usually symbolically representative of the conflict itself.

Hysteria, obsessions, and phobias all shared the same formula and were classified together as the *defense neuropsychoses*. Obsessions represented attachments to symbolic displacements of the objects of earlier psychosexual stages (oral, anal, phallic); phobias embodied the overwhelming fear of such objects, similarly displaced into contemporary symbols.

This revolutionary formulation, elegant for its time and context, begged questions: What is the mechanism that diverts emotion and its energy from conscious to unconscious? How is that energy converted to the observed symptoms? In what part of the mental apparatus is emotion contained? The reader may now see how the accumulation of more clinical experience pushed the model past its limits and forced these questions. In yet another creative leap, Freud produced the structural model, as described in Chapter 1, which addressed these difficulties and expanded the horizon of psychodynamic explanation of psychopathology.

The structural model, introduced in 1923, postulated the presence of id, ego, and superego, allowing the fundamental problems of the topographic model of psychopathology to be addressed. At its most basic, the structural formulation of psychopathology maintains:

- Drive impulses originate in the id.
- As the affects and behavior deriving from these impulses press upon awareness, superego rejects some of them and ego is threatened by their power. The battle among the structures is the essence of psychological *conflict.*
- Ego erects various defensive strategies to contain or divert these undesirable impulses. Most, if not all, of this defensive containment happens unconsciously. Most of the mechanisms employed would be considered irrational by the conscious ego.
- The end result of these defensive distortions of id impulses and drive derivatives is a panoply of symptoms, cognitive, emotional, and/or behavioral.

Thus Fraulein von R.'s circumstances could be more fully explicated: Her desire for her brother-in-law, originating in libidinal id impulses, was rejected by her superego even before it ever reached conscious awareness. Ego contained it first by repression, which only worked temporarily. As the urges persisted just beyond awareness, ego was forced to redirect the libidinal energy through symbolic representation in somatic symptoms.

The expansion of drive theory to include a conflict model allowed psychoanalysis to address many more dimensions of psychopathology, including affect. For Freud and his followers, the primary emotion was anxiety; all others were modifications, displacements, or substitutions. The model of anxiety based in structural theory held that anxiety of one sort is the inevitable result when the influx of energy from any stimulus is greater than what the individual can master. This type of anxiety was labeled *traumatic anxiety;* birth was the prototype for such a stimulus. The growing infant experiences similar sorts of automatic anxiety when he or she is hungry or in pain. Because the ego is still immature, this reflex form of anxiety is almost the only entity in the infant's affective repertoire.

Later, the ego gains the capacity for memory and can connect traumatic, anxiety-provoking events to their surroundings. The infant notices that he or she only gets hungry in the absence of mother; that the dog barks and causes fear. The young ego associates the departure of mother or the presence of the dog with sensations of anxiety and develops the capacity for *signal anxiety*. Even though there is nothing inherently traumatic about the presence of the dog or the absence of the mother, the child has come to associate those signal events with impending anxiety.

Signal anxiety in the more mature ego can deal similarly with internal stimuli, those stemming from unacceptable id impulses. In the presence of a forbidden love object, the wishes of unrestrained libido would be intolerable. The experience of signal anxiety when he or she approaches is weaker and much more manageable. Additionally, it allows the ego to prepare an array of defenses to contain and manage the drive derivatives.

The first and most indispensable tool of the ego in managing anxiety is the defense mechanism of repression. Unacceptable impulses are unconsciously extruded from the ego and returned to the id. But with the impulses goes all their associated energy; so when ego engages in repression, it feeds some of its energy to the id, which then presses its desires all the more powerfully. Too much repression, therefore, promotes the emergence of emotional, cognitive, and/or behavioral pathology. This constellation was named *anxiety neurosis*. Collectively, the earlier-defined defense neuropsychoses (hysteria, obsessions, and phobias) and anxiety neurosis were now labeled as the *psychoneuroses*.

> MR. BROWN acts out a typical "success neurosis." He first identifies with father and attempts to achieve both interpersonal sexual success and external business success. Either achievement would echo the original Oedipal situation; and just on the brink of this success, Oedipal guilt emerges, and he fears the consequence in the form of castration anxiety. As a result, his superego must defeat his id aims rather than allow ego to achieve his goal and put him at risk for retribution.

Paranoia

An early example of the application of this model is in Freud's view of paranoia, drawn from the case of a patient, Daniel S., who maintained a fixed and unshakable belief that his prior psychiatrist was engaged in a plot to change him into woman and abuse him. From his own associations and memories, Daniel painted a picture of a sadistic father who engaged in some very unusual methods of disciplining him. Fearing castration if his father should ever discover

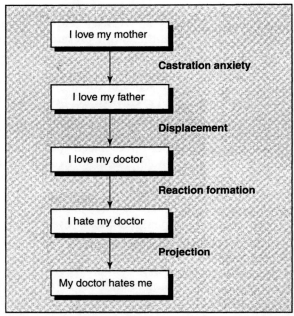

FIGURE 7-1 █ Drive model of paranoia.

his Oedipal urges, Daniel defensively retreated to his father as a love object. This homosexual solution was utterly unacceptable to Daniel's superego and became securely repressed. The intimate relationship with the prior psychiatrist fanned the flames of this desire within his id. He had to deny his love and substitute an imagined hate. That hate for a figure of authority, however, evoked the same fears as Daniel's youthful castration anxiety and led to projection of that hate onto the psychiatrist. (See Figure 7-1.)

As much as this solution put Daniel in jeopardy, it was a preferable compromise to the conscious awareness of his repressed homosexual desires. All other psychopathology mimics, usually with lesser severity, this substitution of a set of psychoneurotic symptoms for conscious awareness of an unacceptable id impulse.

Depression

While Freud focused almost exclusively on anxiety as the primary pathological emotional state, he made a major contribution to the understanding of depression in his 1905 paper, "Mourning and

Melancholia." *Mourning* he defined as the state of experience in which a person has lost a significant love object or abstract representation of such an object and feels sadness about the loss. The emotion is entirely conscious, as is the awareness of the loss, although its meaning may be hidden in the unconscious. (For example, a person who has lost a job may not immediately recognize that the job represents a feeling of potency in the world or a potential source of parental approval. But he or she is consciously aware of feeling sad and consciously connects the sadness to the job loss.)

Melancholia, by contrast, is a much more deep-seated sense of despair, often marked by apathy and pessimism. The object of the sadness may be entirely unavailable to awareness, or the identified loss may be utterly insufficient to justify the degree of distress. In such cases, Freud usually found that there was an unconscious perception of loss of something within the self. The link between the stimulus and the emotional response was suppressed, as was the symbolic significance that linked them. (For example, a woman who strongly but unconsciously identified her boss with her father, and made him the object of unconscious libidinal wishes, might become seriously depressed after the economy forced the company to let her go.) Self-reproach directed toward the representation of that object within the ego is as typical as anger is at the lost object. People who have suffered repeated or intense early losses may be more vulnerable to experiencing this type of depression when other losses occur in adult life. Those with particularly harsh superegos are more susceptible to self-criticism.

Even after a century, the formulation retains validity: Mourning (or grief or bereavement) is a conscious state of sadness linked by the patient to a specific external loss. Melancholia (depression proper in contemporary terminology) is a more profound state of despair in which the loss is perceived as being within the self, and the links are mostly unconscious.

Character Traits

While drive psychology never addressed what are now defined as personality disorders, Freud's followers, particularly Karl Abraham (1877–1925) elucidated character types that represented a persistent, background form of psychopathology. As described in Chapter 1, normal psychosexual development proceeds through stages: oral (first year), anal (1–3 years old), and phallic (3–5 years old). Each entails its own developmental demands. Failure to cope with the demands of any phase can result in *fixation*, an inability to move beyond the characteristics of that stage; stress or stimulus beyond ego's capacity to cope at later points in life can lead to *regression*, a return to an earlier developmental level.

Oral character types are the product of parents who are either too frustrating or too gratifying of oral needs in the first year. These people are overly concerned with the balance between passivity and activity, between dependency and independence. Their thoughts and fantasies are occupied with the need to be nurtured and cared for. Their behavior is characterized by a noteworthy focus on things such as eating and smoking; indulging excess or obsessively limiting, depending on whether the parents were overindulgent or withholding. Overgratified infants become optimistic, contented adults; frustrated infants become pessimistic grown-ups.

Anal character types are the product of parents who cannot help their children through the stage surrounding toilet training and its related tasks. The children's attempts to restrain their bodies' natural anal impulses yield an overconcern with self-control. They grow up to be excessively orderly and interpersonally inflexible. Because, in the symbolic lexicon of drive psychology, feces equates to both dirt and money, anal characters are parsimonious and obsessively neat. However, because this restraint is born of conflict, the underlying impulses frequently break through the repression barrier in episodes or islands of messiness or indulgence.

EGO PSYCHOLOGY

As the structural model allowed psychoanalysts to unfold the mechanisms of a range of affect and pathology, it became clear that id impulses were the driving force behind these phenomena and that superego often counterbalanced it, at a cost of internal conflict. It also became clear that the production of symptoms and their specific relationship to the underlying conflicts was the work of the ego.

Anna Freud, in *The Ego and the Mechanisms of Defense* (1936, revised 1967) put flesh on the bones of the earlier formulations.

She examined the reasons a person might fear direct expression of drives. In some instances, the very strength of the drive threatens to upset the internal harmony of the individual. For example, critical words from a supervisor may trigger murderous derivatives of the aggressive drive, requiring extra energy and creativity on the part of ego, producing paralyzing anxiety. Sometimes the values and standards of the superego are so rigorous that they are threatened by id impulses. For example, a meek and constrained man is taken to a strip show on an out-of-town business trip, his aroused libido triggers massive countermeasures from superego, and he finds his heart in his throat and his concentration impaired for the rest of the trip. And sometimes drives may yield mutually incompatible urges. A classic case of this is the man who experiences intense homosexual and heterosexual desires; each threatens the other and he exhibits the "Don Juan syndrome" of obsessive pursuit of multiple women, with the unconscious aim of submerging the homosexual impulses beneath the volume of heterosexual behavior.

Heinz Hartmann extended Anna Freud's formulations and specified the function of adaptation as the pre-eminent role of the ego. "Fitting together" with the environment is the optimal outcome of successful adaptation. Hartmann was intent on constructing a general psychology and focused almost exclusively on normal development. But there are undeniable implications in his model, elaborated by his followers, about the origins of psychopathology.

Failure to adapt and a resultant inability to fit together, does not necessarily produce pathological affects and behaviors. The inability to adapt may be a product of deficiencies in the environment, abnormalities within the person, or disorders of equilibrium between the two.

Just as in the original Freudian model, anxiety is the first and most important affect experienced by the ego. It appears when id impulses threaten to overwhelm the defenses or as a signal of threat or loss from the environment. Transformation of anxiety into a different, less threatening affect is among the many tools available to ego for mastering it. Commonly, for example, if a person is put into a helpless situation, anxiety may be transformed into anger, which gives the ego more of a sense of potential mastery. In a classic (though by now widely discredited) formulation of depression, when the pressure of aggressive urges threatens to produce anxiety, the ego may turn the aggression inward on the self. Instead of being the anxious purveyor of aggression, the ego is now its depressed victim.

The illuminating elaboration of ego mechanisms in this model yields some ambiguity. The very mechanisms that drive development and support the structure of the ego are the same ones that produce symptoms. In developing a general psychology, the ego psychologists blurred the line between normality and psychopathology. Using this model, it becomes more useful to think of the relevance of adaptive mechanisms to the tasks at hand. The defensive operations that serve to build the ego at age 4, if they do not evolve over time, usually turn out to be maladaptive to living among others as an adult. Furthermore, a defense such as compulsive attention to detail may prevent a father from playing with his children, but may be very adaptive in his work as a surgeon. When defenses, or even symptoms, are integrated with, and acceptable to, the entire personality, they are considered *ego syntonic*. When elements of the personality regard the defense as a source of problems, and wish to be rid of it, it is *ego dystonic*. It is the latter group of defenses that may be defined as symptoms.

OBJECT RELATIONS

MS. GRAY has a limited range of defense mechanisms from which to choose; a consequence of the developmental deficits outlined in prior chapters. She has repressed memories of traumatic episodes in her childhood. She uses splitting to identify others, including boyfriends and therapists, as idealized saviors or as malicious failures. Angered by the therapist's upcoming absence, she regresses and turns her aggression against herself, threatening suicide. More mature mechanisms such as altruism and sublimation appear unavailable to her. While she may have achieved some products of the conflict-free realm of development, she is unable to mobilize them to buffer the effects of environmental stressors and is subject to extreme and unpredictable shifts of emotion.

As object relations theory clarified the role of others (or the internal representation of others) in normal human development, it also undertook to explain psychopathology in similar terms.

Under the broad umbrella of object relations theories, there is a variety of models of affect and psychopathology. Each model is consistent with its underlying theory of development and normal function.

Melanie Klein

Melanie Klein emphasized the role of innate aggression in mental life and defined the paranoid-schizoid and depressive positions of fantasy and emotion. Aggression, no longer just the byproduct of frustration or repressed libido as it had been in Hartmann's model, was now identified as the prime source of guilt and it was identified with prohibited parts of the superego.

Where Freud had identified the primary conflict between drive and reality, Klein saw it as an internal one, between love and hate. For her, ego repudiates the drives not because they conflict with external reality, but because they arouse intolerable feelings inside. Since Klein's infant is born with aggression and hate, and since there is never any love without hate, the child is torn between love and hate, both for self and for (represented) objects. Too immature to accommodate these contradictory feelings with ambivalence, the child experiences a fear of retaliation by the persecutory object (initially, usually the infant's own projections of the parent) and thus feels anxious. The developing ego's first mode of defense is not repression as it was for Freud, but expulsion, an attempt to get rid of the source of anxiety. But in order to protect itself, the ego destroys the object. This sadistic attempt to destroy, however, only generates more anxiety in a vicious cycle. Anxiety is the predominant affect of the paranoid position. What Klein labeled as the "schizoid" component of this position is the splitting of aggressive impulses out of the self and onto the objects by projection. As terrifying as this formulation may be, it is preferable to the fear of annihilation by one's own destructive impulses.

If the child is unable to transcend this immature constellation, he or she retains those core feelings of persecutory expectation and fearful tension. Klein herself was not specific about what circumstances either facilitated or inhibited this transition, but her successors added more precision to her model. Most children will advance to the depressive position, where they love their mothers and seek to introject them so they can provide protection. But the aggression never disappears, so the introjected maternal object remains vulnerable to the same attack. The child is now tormented by anxiety over the consequences of his or her intense feelings of sadism. The ego now has the maturity to defend against this anxiety by attempting reparations; now there is no hate without love.

MS. WHITE is caught between hate and love for both her husband and her children. Hungry for affection and intimacy with Mr. White, she is burdened by her anger with him for intruding on her in his premature retirement. Her sense of abandonment by her children threatens her maternal love for them. Just below her awareness, she is feeling guilty for having such thoughts and fears they will destroy the very objects of her love.

Most of adulthood is characterized by this tension. Under the best of circumstances, the conflict between aggression and libido foster growth of the ego. The ego develops the capacity for ambiguity and for healing through mourning lost objects. But when aggression generates excessive anxiety, libido is mobilized to oppose it, and the balance becomes fixed at that stage. Anxiety is focused on the injury done to the object by one's love and hate or on the fear of loss of the object. Alternatively, or additionally, guilt can arise from responsibility for harm done to the object by one's aggressive fantasies. The mechanism of splitting may be mobilized even in the depressive position as the child constructs good objects to contain gratification and bad objects to contain rage.

Margaret Mahler

Although Mahler focused much more on the processes of normal development, her specification of the characteristics of the "average expectable environment" bore implications for object relations models of psychopathology. Particularly, she noted that the unconscious aspects of the mother influenced the success of all stages of development from the symbiotic phase onward. She noted, for example that parental attitudes toward locomotion directly affect the child's success in achieving this capacity. It followed, then, that parental attitudes of overprotection or apathy would inhibit this vital step in ego development.

Particularly important is maternal anxiety. The nervous or dissatisfied mother is unable to provide a successful partner for the baby's symbiotic needs. The child may get vegetative satisfaction but will not connect it with the gratification of emotional needs.

Such a child will grow up with "affect hunger" and pursue relationships later in life with unfulfillable expectations and predictable disappointment.

W.R.D. Fairbairn

Our understanding of Fairbairn's views of pathogenesis is limited by his minimal writings and must be gleaned mostly by implication. At the core, Fairbairn maintained that all portions of the ego are tied to objects. It is, in fact, the primary function of ego to relate to objects. All psychopathology derives from the ego's futile efforts to perpetuate archaic ties to internal objects.

When early relationships fail to provide nurturance for the young child, the ego establishes object images inside itself which function as substitutes for the depriving real objects. Where normal development revolves around relationships with real others, psychopathology revolves around relationships with these imaginary internal images. The greater the difference between the compensatory internal objects and the real external ones, the greater the distortions that characterize the pathological world view. Aggression, not a primary motivator as it was for Klein, is instead the result of frustration with primary objects.

D. W. Winnicott

Winnicott's path of normal development was vitally dependent on an appropriately responsive parent. Very early, the infant required near perfect mothering, and subsequently he or she needed a mother who would respond with exquisite sensitivity to normal frustrations. His model of psychopathology relies on this view, and describes two types of pathogenic maternal failures:

- the inability to bring the infant's hallucinatory wishes to reality, and
- interference with the quiescent states necessary for formation of the early self.

To the child, such failures represent a frightening disruption of the continuity of personal existence, since he or she is yet unable to perceive self as separate from mother. This disruption yields fragmentations of experience, which then coalesce into the true and false selves. (See Chapter 5.) The false self evolves and grows in order to comply with the failings of the mother. The strivings of the true self are repressed in proportion to parental failings.

Mental health for Winnicott was defined by the integrity and spontaneity of the self, so psychopathology reflected a distortion and constraint in the expression of the self. Since the false self must rely heavily on cognitive operations to determine how to comply with the inadequate mother, the ascendancy of the false self is manifest in an overactive mind in which cognition is separated from genuine emotion.

Winnicott devised his own scheme of diagnosis grounded in this model. Disorders were of three types:

- Pre-self disorders, characterized by breakdown within the most primitive sets of object relations. Such conditions included psychosis, schizoid conditions and borderline states.
- Depressive disorders were Kleinian problems with the conflict between love and hate in the internal object world.
- Neuroses were manifestations of classical Freudian conflict.

Over time, Winnicott reclassified the Freudian neurotics as belonging to a small class of very healthy individuals, because the existence of a classical neurosis required the presence of an intact and continuous self, which in turn reflected healthy parenting. He also categorized Kleinian depressive disorders as characteristic of the majority of presumably normal people struggling with non-pathologic emotions. As a result, he was left maintaining that all psychopathology fell into the category of pre-self disorders, and all resulted from parental failings.

Otto Kernberg

Kernberg's information base was a population of severely disturbed individuals with borderline and narcissistic personality disorders. His contribution to the theory of psychopathology was a detailed description of the inner workings of such primitive personalities, and this theory is entirely consistent with his model of pre-Oedipal development.

Affect in his model, as presented in Chapter 4, is not a product of the ego; rather it is a characteristic of the primary relational experience with the significant object. It is a feature of the shared field of object and self. Turning the older model on its head, Kernberg postulates that psychic structures and even the drives are themselves determined by the emotional coloration of very early experiences. Under ideal circumstances, the nature of the object and the quality of the affect lead to a smooth development of properly functioning mental structures.

In his dealings with primitive personalities, he observed the consequences of abnormal developmental contexts. If the emotional environment of early experiences is perceived as much more unpleasant than pleasant, then "good" object representations cannot outweigh and master "bad" ones. In the presence of such an imbalance, the primitive split between good and bad experiences and representations is never overcome, and the merger that is necessary for a robust ego is never complete. The *splitting* that is a normal function of the early mind is never abandoned, and the consequences are profound.

The borderline adult continues to split good and bad experiences absolutely. From moment to moment, others in the environment are perceived as either all good, capable of providing love, comfort, and fulfillment; or all bad, depriving, withholding, and malicious. Such splitting prevents a person from viewing another as simply decent or flawed. Such overvaluation and depreciation alternate rapidly and in the extreme, leading to corollary vacillations of emotional state, from excited to euphoric, and in attitude, from love to hate. Since the image of the self is a product of object relations, such a person suffers from intense and dichotomous views of himself or herself. The borderline or severely narcissistic individual cannot see himself or herself as a constant, singular individual who can be trusted to feel or act in predictable ways. Each moment is an unprecedented, and dangerous, adventure.

MS. GRAY behaves in a way consistent with Kernberg's borderline level of personality organization. Her early experiences were laden with bad affective colorations, and she was thus unable to integrate her object experiences. In the present, she lacks a consistent view of herself or of the objects in her environment. Splitting characterizes her function. She experiences each new relationship, whether with a boyfriend or a therapist, in a positive light and holds out high expectations. These are inevitably disappointed and are replaced in a flash with negative perceptions and overtly aggressive behavior. Not only do the others in her world shift rapidly from good to bad, but so does her image of herself. Her pursuit of calming through drugs and alcohol is an attempt to dull the pain of her self-directed aggressive impulses, and one that is doomed to failure.

Further complicating matters, the splitting is not just between good and bad experiences and impressions, but also between mental functions. Kernberg noted from his clinical work that borderline patients would act on impulse with no evident awareness of the emotion and ideation associated with the behavior. When he would point out the correlation, his patients would typically blandly acknowledge the cognitive validity of his observations, but would be unable to incorporate it in a meaningful or emotional way. This splitting of experience from structure impairs the individual's capacity to learn from experience, either in therapy or in life. The disordered behavior that characterizes the lives of borderline individuals is a consequence of their reactivity to environmental events, unbuffered by internal affective constancy, and by their complementary search for stability and fulfillment in the wrong places.

SELF PSYCHOLOGY

Since self psychology rejects both the drives and the psychic structures of drive, ego, and object relations psychologies, it stands to reason that the self-psychological formulation of psychopathology would bear little resemblance to the nosology of the other models. Indeed, self psychologists use the label "selfobject relational disorders" to identify psychopathology. If all psychological development is based on selfobject functions, then derailed development is describable in terms of faulty selfobject experiences.

Loosely, self psychology lists types of disorders in a ranking of severity:

- Psychoses exhibit extremes of severely absent self-soothing and cohesion.
- Borderline states are characterized by permanent weakness or chaotic organization of the nuclear self.
- Narcissistic disorders, including narcissistic personality disorders and the less-severe narcissistic behavior disorders, are less intense and dysfunctional than borderline states. They are marked by moderate instability of mood and self-defeating behavior.
- Psychoneuroses, characterized by the same symptoms as those of the classical models, are a special variant of narcissistic disorder.

From the self psychological perspective, disorders are characterized not by their phenomenology, but by their etiology. Symptoms, whether emotional, cognitive, or behavioral, are the manifestations of a particular deficit of selfobject function, filtered through temperament and contemporary experience. (Remember in the ensuing discussions that "selfobject" refers not to a person but to a selfobject function or experience.)

Because there is no ego, id, or superego and because there are no drives, there is no place in this model for conflict between drives or among structures. The word "conflict" has no place in the self psychology lexicon. Instead, because the nuclear self is the product of selfobjects, all problems are the result of selfobject *deficits*. This distinction between conflict and deficit is probably the single biggest difference between the self-psychological model of pathology and all others. Healthy mental function is the product of a cohesive nuclear self. When that cohesion is threatened, by external events, internal thoughts, or maladaptive perceptions, what we observe as symptoms are the *breakdown products* of the unstable nucleus attempting to right itself.

Since mirroring selfobjects nurture the pole of the grandiose self, which in turn fosters self-esteem regulation, enjoyment, and the pursuit of goals and purposes, it follows that a deficit in selfobject mirroring will yield instability of self-esteem, lack of pleasure, and weak ambitions. At the other pole, the idealizable selfobject allows for the establishment and growth of the idealized parental imago, which is responsible for self-soothing, regulation of feelings, the capacity for enthusiasm, and devotion to ideals. Inadequate objects of idealization predispose to instability of mood, apathy, and a narrow, self-centered outlook. The result of such deficits, or imbalances between the poles of the nuclear self, depends on factors such as the severity of the deficit, the developmental stage at which it was experienced, the duration of the deficit, and the compensatory resources available in the environment.

At the least severe end of the spectrum, the psychoneuroses are the outcome of deficits experienced during the Oedipal stage of development, i.e., ages 4 to 6, at a time when the child is becoming aware of genital sensations and is capable of feeling guilty. If the deficit is in the area of the grandiose self, an adult under a stress that resonates with his or her deficits (e.g., a divorce), might experience self-doubt, anhedonia, and limited new activities.

MR. BROWN had an idealizable selfobject in his father, although his mother was deficient in her abilities to provide those experiences. Neither parent offered much in the way of mirroring. Mr. Brown's bipolar self is thus skewed in the direction of narcissistic needs. His pattern has been to pursue aims reflecting the paternal ideals he internalized, but to fall short because of his narcissistic deficits. Failing to receive the mirroring in adulthood that he has lacked since childhood, he repeatedly trips himself up before achieving success. While he is able to regulate his affect fairly reliably, he has less success in regulating his self-esteem, and his presenting symptoms represent fragmentation products of his selfobject pursuits. Further, the imbalance in his bipolar self deprives him of the optimal adult capacity for empathy, contributing to the unsatisfying nature of his relationships with those closest to him.

Narcissistic disorders are more pervasive and detrimental. They result from more persistent and severe deficits than those yielding psychoneuroses. Here, a deficit in the function of the idealizable selfobject might cause an adult to become anxious and self-centered. Addictive behaviors or perversions may be mobilized to shore up the selfobject deficits.

Borderline states, resulting from severe, early, and ongoing deficits in selfobject function, usually at both poles, require the constant mobilization of complex defenses for psychic survival. Schizoid attitudes or histrionic style may serve the function of keeping contemporary relationships shallow to avoid repetition of the harm from the early noxious ones. Paranoid strategies may allow the person to disown blame for intolerable feeling states. Instability of mood and self-esteem, chaos of self-image and external behavior, are the norm. Compared to persons with narcissistic selfobject disorders, borderline individuals have a much more feeble capacity for reality testing and objectivity.

Learning points

- Drive psychology best describes the classical neurotic disorders, including anxiety neurosis, neurotic depression, and obsessive-compulsive neurosis. It does so in terms of the defenses that must be mounted to prevent id drives from emerging into awareness.

- Ego psychology explains pathology as a failure to adapt to the interpersonal environment and uses the defense mechanisms to specify the nature of individual affects and psychopathological conditions.
- Object relations theories, constituting a more divergent group than the other schools, offer a range of explanations of affect and pathology.
  - Melanie Klein focuses on the role of aggression and the struggle between love and hate.
  - Margaret Mahler sees adult conditions as reflections of early problems with separation and individuation.
  - D.W. Winnicott puts the struggle between the true self and the false self at the core of adult problems.
  - Otto Kernberg most particularly defined borderline psychopathology, noting particularly the persistence of infantile splitting.
- Self psychology traces adult pathology to deficiencies in mirroring and/or idealizable selfobject functions and identifies comparable defects in the capacities for regulating affect and/or self-esteem.

RECOMMENDED READINGS

Fairbairn WRD. A revised psychopathology of the psychoses and psychoneuroses. *Int J Psycho-Anal.*1941;22:250–279.

Fisher S, Greenberg RP. *Freud Scientifically Reappraised: Testing the Theories and Therapy.* New York: John Wiley & Sons, 1996.

Rangell L. Affects. In: Moore BE, Fine B, eds. *Psychoanalysis: The Major Concepts.* New Haven, CT: Yale University Press, 1995:381–391.

Siegel AM. *Heinz Kohut and the Psychology of the Self.* London: Routledge, 1996.

Spezzano C. *Affect in Psychoanalysis: A Clinical Synthesis.* London: The Analytic Press, 1993.

Stein R. *Psychoanalytic Theories of Affect.* New York: Praeger, 1991.

Therapy and Cure I:
Drive and Ego Psychologies

"Health is a state of complete physical, mental and social well-being, and not merely the absence of disease or infirmity."
—*from Constitution of the World Health Organization*

LEARNING OBJECTIVES

The reader will be able to:

1. Relate the drive and ego models of therapy to their respective models of development and pathogenesis.
2. List the pertinent questions for each model of therapy.
3. Outline the evolution of drive theories of cure.
4. Compare the therapeutic aims of drive and ego psychologies.
5. Define the types of patients for whom each form of therapy is appropriate.

All the theories of psychodynamics were derived and elaborated by clinicians. The questions they sought to answer were those generated by the challenging problems of psychoanalysis and psychotherapy. Our examination of the theories thus concludes with an outline of the therapeutic implications of each of the models in this chapter and the next.

Each theory of the mind, as we have seen, leads to a different set of conclusions about what normal mental function should be and about what goes wrong in various mental disorders. It follows that each model of therapy subscribes to the same assumptions about normality and pathology, and each seeks to use the therapy to set right whatever has gone wrong.

DRIVE THEORY

The drive model posits the existence of libidinal and aggressive drives that fuel all mental activity. Mental content may be unconscious, preconscious, or fully conscious, and the execution of drive activity is mediated by the three structures. Id is the most primitive structure, seeking immediate and unqualified gratification of drive hungers. Superego is the societally driven structure that establishes ideals of behavior and punishes transgressions. Ego is the navigating and executive structure, mobilizing motor and cognitive powers to fulfill id desires by manipulating the environment or by performing internal mental operations to attenuate the drives. Foremost among these latter measures is the array of defense mechanisms that allow ego to keep id, superego, and reality in some dynamic balance. Psychopathology results when drive urges overwhelm the ability of the various structures to gratify or contain them. The same defenses that serve the ends of id and ego can also cause emotional distress and behavioral dysfunction.

In giving birth to psychoanalysis, Sigmund Freud, flush with his early successes in treating hysteria, assumed that alleviation from symptoms would come directly and simply from awareness of their unconscious origins. From the narrow range of his early exposures, he concluded that all hysteria was the outcome of prior trauma. Every life experience, he reasoned, is accompanied by a quota of emotion, which is normally released in a nonsymptomatic way. Traumatic experiences are accompanied by excess emotion, which cannot be discharged through normal means. Therapy required "abreaction," the reawakening and release of memories and emotions in the present. When met with the verbal responses of the analyst, such abreaction would not only release the "strangulated" affect but would also give a conscious, rational framework for the pathogenic memories and permit correction by association with more adaptive thoughts. Working purely within the topographic model, his goal was "to make the unconscious

conscious." By recovering memories under hypnosis, then later by encouraging patients to delve into their memories without censorship ("free association"), he relied on the recovery of repressed memories and ideas to cure neurotic symptoms.

Before long, it became apparent that pure awareness was insufficient for most patients. They would distort memories and perceptions; they would substitute new symptoms for old ones; and they would repeat pathological patterns of behavior. He saw that the symptoms were not merely the result of constitutional weakness, but comprised a particular effort of the mind to deal with intolerable clusters of memory, thought, and emotion by revising or expelling them. As the subtleties of repression and distortion revealed themselves in analysis, Freud found that he needed further to interpret the meanings of symptoms. As the structural model evolved and analysts became aware of the multiplicity of maneuvers and tools available to the ego, the aim of therapy shifted. The analyst now sought to understand the meanings of symptoms and to determine motivations. The key element of therapy was not just awareness but interpretation. Said Freud, "Where id was, there ego shall be." (See Table 8-1.)

Change in symptoms, behavior, emotion, and even personality could result from this self-awareness when the patient became:

- Aware of unconscious conflicts and defenses
- Aware of the origin of these unconscious elements
- Able to overcome these conflicts and defenses consciously, and
- Able to organize thought, feeling, and action to satisfy drives in a manner appropriate to reality.

The achievement of these simple ends was confounded by several factors. Simple encouragement did not always bring unconscious memories to the fore. Repression was a powerful force,

TABLE 8-1	*Sigmund Freud's Evolving Goals of Psychoanalysis*
1886–1905	Making the unconscious conscious
1905–1914	Working through transference and other resistances
1915–1923	"Where id was, there ego shall be."
1923–1929	Promoting optimal ego functioning

and the defenses obscured the analyst's vision of the unconscious mind. Furthermore, the patient's distortions were not limited to alterations of memory, but affected how he or she perceived others in his or her life, including the analyst. Freud and his early colleagues noted that patients recognized their analysts as characters from their pasts, playing out on them the manifestations of drive-based wishes and fears. Because old patterns were transferred into the present, this pattern became known as "transference."

Sigmund Freud had the creativity to perceive resistance and transference as more than just impediments to therapy but also as a field of investigation on the path to cure. Since brute force of persuasion could rarely penetrate the resistances, the best alternative was to analyze the resistances themselves. In doing so, the analyst obtained a richly textured picture of the workings of the ego by observing its defenses in operation. Even more so, the analysis of transference yielded tremendous insights. As drive urges, ego defenses, and superego fright were manifested in vivo, the analyst could deal with otherwise unconscious material directly in the consulting room. By observing the patient's responses to environmental stimuli, the analyst could determine the motivation and meaning in the pattern of defense, resistance, and transference. When the analyst does not behave like the original object, the analytic patient becomes aware of the discrepancy, disrupting the automatic patterns to which the patient has become accustomed, and change becomes possible.

In the formal process of psychoanalysis, the patient does more than play out symptoms in the transference. He or she recreates the totality of the pathogenic neurotic conflict within the analytic setting, including the analyst as a figure in that constellation. This configuration is termed the *transference neurosis* and is critical to the success of a classical psychoanalysis. The analysand's attention shifts away from exclusive focus on events and personalities outside the analysis and directs itself toward the person of the analyst and the environment of the consulting room. The analyst allows these perceptions, complaints, and demands to unfold—an often uncomfortable passage for both parties—offering interpretations of parallels to the pathogenic situation. Since these interpretations now strike "closer to home" than those about external circumstances (after all, the party offering the interpretations is in fact the primary object of the patient's distortions), the resistances are denser and more complex. By the same token, when they have been absorbed and implemented (see below), their power is profound, since the interpretations have been offered and the changes made in vivo, and the patient has come through the experience of understanding his or her neurosis from the inside out, solving its riddles with the aid of an active party to the conflicts.

When an interpretation is offered, a repressed conflict is mobilized and enters consciousness, if only partially. This revelation induces anxiety, which both mobilizes further defenses and also drives the pursuit of change through the analytic process. As the patient comes to perceive the differences between the transference object and the original object, cognitive mastery makes the energy available to the ego. True structural change occurs as ego is strengthened by the energy that was formerly connected to repressed drives and conflicts.

 MS. GRAY's therapist offered the speculation that the patient longed for the affection of her father, even though she was frightened by his brutality. She repeatedly entered into relationships with alcoholic and abusive men in an attempt to enact the childhood fantasy of union with her father. Ms. Gray rejected the interpretation at first, scoffing at the idea she could foster any lingering attraction to her father. At the next session, she reported that she had had another fight with Michael, admittedly partly at her own provocation. With prompting and inquiry by the therapist, she could acknowledge that, in the aftermath, she felt much as she had in her youth after one of her father's alcoholic outbursts: helpless and frightened but also longing for healing affection from her adversary. The therapist's aim was to bring into conscious awareness a derivative of infantile libidinal drive, which Ms. Gray could eventually use to foster more adaptive ego capacities.

One product of the Oedipal phase of development is the emergence of the superego. As described in Chapter 7, superego plays a major role in many types of pathology in the drive model, since it opposes id at almost every turn and forces ego to devise often neurotic compromises. From the beginning of an analysis, superego blocks the flow of free associations and triggers ego to suppress the memories, feelings, and thoughts underlying the problems being addressed. Superego similarly inhibits awareness of transference feelings, forcing ego to devise elaborate distortions of id's wishes. It is therefore an early mandate for the analyst to help relax the constraints of the superego. He or she does so by modeling a more benign attitude toward pathogenic impulses than the patient's superego, by interpreting superego restrictions, by directly encouraging free association, and by highlighting transference manifestations. Analyzing the origin of superego ideals and limitations, of course, leads directly to analysis of the Oedipus complex.

A single flash of insight was never enough to affect a cure or anything more than transient remission of symptoms. Real change required that the patient take the explanations offered by the analyst, put them in place in the events of the world, and try to replace distortions and defenses with conscious ego adaptations. In the process called "working through," the patient would engage in repeated exercises of newfound insight to achieve long-lasting relief and personal growth. One of Freud's essential papers on the therapeutic process was entitled, "Remembering, repeating and working through" (1914). Over the course of analysis, a patient would enter because he or she was *repeating* old and repressed patterns; analysis allowed him or her to *remember*; and conscious awareness afforded the opportunity for him or her to *work through* the conflict and adopt more adaptive perceptions and responses.

The structural model maintained that drive energy was the content of the id and that psychopathology resulted from conflicts between unconscious drives' urges and both reality and the superego. Science at the turn of the 20th century had already described much about the workings of the conscious mind. The early analysts had the most to contribute in their understandings of the unconscious. And the drive model of therapy focused primarily on the id.

In analyzing the symptoms created by the ego and its defense mechanisms, analysts guided by drive theory ask:

- What drive urge is being expressed?
- What unconscious ideas are forcing the drive wishes to be repressed?
- What defenses is the ego using to deal with the urges?
- How do the defenses themselves reflect the id's drives?
- What compromise is ego maintaining among drive wish, defense, and reality?
- How effective are the defenses?
- How are these patterns being manifest in the transference?

The answers to these questions constitute the content of the analyst's interpretations. In the earliest days, interpretations were quite didactic and authoritative. As decades passed, analysts adapted their style to accommodate emotion as much as thought, but the primary focus remains to identify the derivatives of the primitive drives that are fueling the current problems, to bring them to the fore, and to replace unconscious repetition of symptoms with conscious choice of response and initiative. The focus on pathogenesis in early life experiences has grown. More attention has been paid to the role of superego; by contrast with the punitive superego of the patient's transference, the analyst allows a more forgiving superego to develop, diminishing a major source of conflict and anxiety.

The turmoil of the Oedipus complex and its resolution are probably the most frequent objects of attention from the drive-conflict psychoanalyst. Since this period defines the crystallization of the essential psychic structures, the therapist pursues the repressed longings, the memories of parental response, the child's reactions and accommodations, and the adult residua of all these processes. Since the persistence of unresolved Oedipal conflicts necessarily breeds conflict among the structures id, ego, and superego, the analyst is obliged to help the patient achieve resolution. Acknowledgment of libidinal strivings toward the opposite-sex parent and aggressive urges toward the same-sex parent are brought into consciousness. The pressure and tension required to maintain the repression of this content is released for ego to use in diminishing the fear of reprisal from the superego and in fulfilling drive wishes in less symptomatic ways.

The drive model assumes the existence of fully formed structures id, ego, and superego. Treatment based on it requires not only extraordinary motivation but also an ability (on the patient's part) to distance oneself from the irrational products of mental activity in order to observe and analyze them. In technical terms, there must be a strong enough *observing ego* to separate from and modify the *experiencing ego*. Accordingly, the patients most suitable for therapy in this model are those with the classic "neurotic" symptoms such as conversion disorders and performance anxiety, as well as those with moderate levels of affective distress such as dysthymic disorder and generalized anxiety disorder.

Two rules of psychoanalysis enable the patient to uncover the material underlying his or her problems, and the analyst to offer corrective interventions:

> The *fundamental rule* of psychoanalysis is to "say what comes to mind," without editing, revision, or refinement.

■ The *rule of abstinence* prohibits the analyst from gratifying the analysand's wishes.

The aim of the fundamental rule is to overcome by conscious intent the primary defense of repression. Without it, there could be no free association. But if defenses could be conquered by simple force of will, there would be no need for the difficult process of analysis or depth psychotherapy. Consequently much of the analysis is spent detecting and undoing ego's schemes to circumvent the fundamental rule.

The rule of abstinence is necessary to allow transference fantasies and desires to present themselves. The analyst does not dispense coffee, advice, or hugs. He or she typically says much less than the patient. Further, the analyst attempts to remain as anonymous as possible, revealing little about himself or herself outside the context of each patient's individual analysis. (Anonymity is vital in principle but rarely achievable in reality.)

EGO PSYCHOLOGY

Where drive psychology views all pathology originating in id drives and their derivatives, ego psychology pays more attention to the ego's role in managing the drives. People bring to their therapists problems of emotion, thought, and behavior, all of which are functions of the ego. In this model, even though the drives are still active in the id, the symptoms requiring attention are the products of ego's attempts to adapt, accommodate, and master. Before the drives can be addressed, it is necessary to analyze and correct the ego's malfunctions, particularly its defense mechanisms.

At its core, ego psychology maintains the same therapeutic philosophy as drive psychology. Unconscious processes of the psychic structures must be brought into awareness and their origins must be analyzed. Those processes that generate distress can then be replaced with more conscious choices. The primary difference in the ego-psychological approach is the level of focus on defenses and other modes of adaptation. Modification of drives may subsequently be attempted, but is not mandatory. Awareness of drive urges is a tool for comprehending ego functions, not an end in itself.

While this difference may seem like a minor distinction in depth of focus, it hinges on a substantial difference between id and ego. Because id's operations remain almost completely repressed, its nature is hidden and it can only be understood by indirect inference and assumption. Ego, on the other hand, operates more largely in the realm of the conscious and preconscious. Even its unconscious operations generate observable consequences that can be directly reflected and interpreted.

The most commonly observed consequence of ego dysfunction, of course, is anxiety. The ego-psychological therapist is constantly attentive to signals of anxiety. These signals may be evident in the patient's stories about life outside the therapy or in the transference. He or she identifies the anxiety promptly and focuses with the patient on its context. Identifying the emotional state with precision, the pair can examine the defense mechanisms at work.

In the exploration of anxiety and its related affects and behavior, the important questions include:

- What defenses are operating against the drives?
- How effective are they?
- How rigid or flexible are they?
- What is the range of defense mechanisms available?
- What affects are provoking the defensive operations?

Beyond identifying the defense mechanisms, the ego psychologists investigated and explained the origins of the ego. Hartmann, in the earliest iterations of the model, described the emergence of ego from the undifferentiated matrix by way of adaptation to the environment, and he further described the conflict-free areas of ego development. As a result the model of pathogenesis includes not just malfunction in the structure ego but also deficiencies in its very formation. Consequently, the analyst asking the questions above may find that the responses only beg further ones, such as:

- What tools of adaptation have failed to develop abnormally, or at all?
- What areas of the conflict-free sphere are inadequately developed?
- What factors in the environment shaped the maladaptive or inadequate development of the ego?

From the answers to these queries comes the content of the therapeutic interventions. The therapist connects the disturbing affect to the defense mechanisms that produce it. Since the defenses are conceived as modes of adaptation, the typical ego-psychological interpretation identifies the original adaptive effort behind the ego operation, the reasons for its mobilization in a different context, and the negative consequences of that mobilization. The first step in recovery is for the patient to recognize the incompatibility of the automatic defense mechanism to the current situation.

Working through is not only as important as it is in the drive model, but takes place at the level of ego operations. Having arrived at an awareness of the poor fit between prior defenses and contemporary needs, the patient will ideally try new mechanisms consciously and will inevitably mobilize others unconsciously. Over the course of the therapy, patient and therapist can examine the beneficial and deleterious outcomes of different modes of defense and response, ultimately settling on those that work best.

MR. BROWN's therapist identified the early adaptive function of some of his defensive operations: Identification with father protected him against feelings of both shame and inferiority. Stopping short of achievements protected him against feelings of guilt and brought him closer to mother's embrace. At the time these maneuvers were devised, they served their purposes adequately. But as Mr. Brown grew into adulthood, their cost exceeded their benefits. Mr. Brown was able to see that anxiety and isolation were the price of using old methods in contemporary settings. The therapist anticipated that the course of therapy would involve Mr. Brown's considering and experimenting with alternative defensive constellations and weighing their psychic and interpersonal costs and benefits.

As described in Chapter 3, ego psychology takes a more dynamic view of ongoing development than does drive psychology, and this philosophy offers further avenues for intervention. The therapist who endorses a longitudinal developmental model, like those of Erikson or Vaillant, may reflect to the patient how different elements of ego functioning are more or less adaptive at different stages of maturity. Identifying the life crisis reflected in a current problem, for example, directs the therapist to the stage in life when that crisis is usually most active. He or she can explain to the patient the adaptive purpose of the mode of ego operating at that time, and why it is being mobilized at a later stage. Recognizing that the life crises never disappear allows both therapist and patient to approach their appearance "out of time" with less pathological labeling.

 The therapist was impressed with the life-stage issues with which MS. WHITE was struggling. Bearing in mind the relevant crisis of generativity versus self-absorption, he encouraged her to elaborate on the meaning that motherhood played in her sense of identity. "It made me feel useful. I was happy knowing that I was contributing to their well-being." With the therapist's guidance, she explained that she felt she was no longer contributing, since her children were all independent. The therapist asked her to consider whether their independence was itself a measure of her contribution. "I guess it's true, they wouldn't be able to be on their own if I hadn't done well for them in the past. I should be proud of that, shouldn't I?"

Further, she was able to accept the therapist's invitation to identify other avenues for obtaining the same sort of gratification. "I'll have the opportunity to be a grandmother, and I can tell from what we've been discussing that I need to keep my fingers out of my children's parenting. One of my friends asked me to join her on the county's literacy council. That could give me a similar kind of satisfaction."

Hartmann introduced the notion of the conflict-free sphere of development. In therapy, this idea expands the available opportunities. Mechanisms that were previously seen only as defenses can now be seen as positive products of development. The therapist is obliged to investigate these mental capabilities, since they are readily available to the patient for use in situations where the automatic mechanisms are maladaptive. Even when a mechanism has been mobilized originally in a defensive maneuver, it can gain a life of its own, and it can be owned and used by the patient in a nonpathological manner. For example, a weakling who develops precocious verbal capacities as a youngster may exercise and magnify them throughout development long past when they are needed to fend off bullies. This sphere can be exploited in therapy as a valid source of self-esteem and a tool for adaptation, not simply as a pathological residue of early anxiety.

The objects in the world of ego psychology are not as faceless as they are in drive theory, and the therapist aims to specify the nature of particular objects in the patient's world in order to increase the precision of the interpretations. Since father and mother are acknowledged to have their own particular features, patient and therapist can examine how one teacher evokes memories of a particular element of father and how another boss reflects relevant characteristics of mother. The ego operations involved in each relationship can be defined with considerable precision and the links unbound and reworked as they are for defense mechanisms in general.

The acknowledgment of the individuality of objects then has relevance to the nature of transference interventions in ego psychology. The therapist is not the blank screen of drive psychology, but an individual who cannot help but bring personal features to the interaction. The patient's unconscious perceptions and responses are not independent of the therapist's nature and behavior. Instead, they are interpreted in the context of the patient's specific perception of the therapist and/or the therapist's words and actions. The role of transference interpretations in ego psychology is just as important as it is in drive psychology but is carved with a sharper tool.

Like drive psychology, ego psychology requires the collaboration of the ego for therapy to proceed. But the model posits ego elements present from a very early age, and almost none of the ego theorists draws a sharp line of therapeutic availability at the Oedipal transition. Thus, patients may be suitable for psychodynamic therapy for problems originating in pre-Oedipal stages. Furthermore, since the objects in the ego world have greater specificity, problems of interpersonal relationships are a more fitting focus for therapy than they were before the model developed. Consequently, ego-psychological therapy is just as workable for patients with the classical neurotic conditions fitting for drive theory but can also be more broadly applied. Patients with more severe levels of depression or anxiety than those appropriate for drive-based therapy can avail themselves of ego-psychological treatment. Patients with chronic or recurrent interpersonal difficulties can make use of the model. And it can be applied in patients with personality-based pathology of moderate enough severity that some level of observing ego can be mobilized more often than not, i.e., most patients with avoidant, dependent, and obsessive-compulsive personality disorders, and some of those with narcissistic and histrionic personality disorders. Most patients with severe narcissistic personality disorders and those with borderline personality disorders benefit less from therapy based solely in ego psychology.

Learning points

■ As the topographic model was augmented by the dual-drive theory and the structural model, drive theory's therapeutic aims evolved from simply "making the unconscious conscious" to promoting optimal ego functioning.
■ Resistance and transference are opportunities for analytic understanding and therapeutic intervention.
■ Drive theory aims at defining and altering the unconscious drives within the id; ego psychology aims at affecting the defenses and other ego functions which are more accessible to conscious awareness.
■ Ego psychology targets not only defenses in conflict, but also elements of the conflict-free sphere of development. Longitudinal models of development allow for interventions specific to life stage issues.

RECOMMENDED READINGS

Blanck G, Blanck R. *Ego Psychology: Theory and Practice*. 2nd ed. New York: Columbia University Press, 1994.
Loewald HW. On the therapeutic action of psycho-analysis. *Int J Psychoanal*. 1960;41:16–33.
Meissner WW. *Freud and Psychoanalysis*. Notre Dame, IN: University of Notre Dame Press, 2000.
Nersessian E., Kopff RG, Jr. *Textbook of Psychoanalysis*. Washington, D.C.: American Psychiatric Press, 1996.
Polansky N. *Integrated Ego Psychology*. New York: Aldine Pub. Co., 1982.

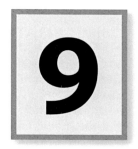

Therapy and Cure II:
The Relational Psychologies

"To love oneself is the beginning of a lifelong romance."
—Oscar Wilde

LEARNING OBJECTIVES

The reader will be able to:

1. List the therapeutic principles common to all major schools of object relations.
2. Define the differences in focus among the major schools of object relations.
3. Describe the curative potential of transference in object relations and self psychologies.
4. Outline the cycle of disruption and restoration in self-psychological therapy.

D rive and ego psychologies are essentially one-person systems and conceptualize therapy as the correction of errors or the repair of injuries within that self-contained system. The relational theories, i.e., the object relations schools and self psychology, view development and psychopathology as creations of an interpersonal environment. It follows that they would have very different philosophies about the curative process of psychotherapy, and the types of interventions that are mandated.

OBJECT RELATIONS

As noted in Chapter 5, although the object relations theories are best known for their differences, they have more in common. While the specifics of intervention and therapeutic style vary across object relations theories, many fundamentals of therapeutic philosophy and the curative process are shared by all of them. Therapeutic principles common to all object relations theories include these:

- Since the patient's problems are relational in origin and nature, cure comes through rectification of perceptions of, and relationships with, others.
- Identification, elaboration, and understanding of emotional states are necessary for the therapeutic process.
- Interventions, especially interpretations, not only convey information, but also convey an interpersonal message and influence the dyadic exchange.
- The patient brings his or her relational patterns into the therapy and these are mobilized in the transference. The transference is also substantially and specifically influenced by the therapist's conduct and communication.
- The patient–therapist interaction has therapeutic potential that transcends the power of interpretations alone.
- Cure is achieved when the patient is released from irresistible repetition of old and maladaptive patterns of perceiving and relating and is free to choose modes fitting to his or her current circumstances.

Comparisons with the one-person psychologies of the drive and ego models highlight the tenets that characterize object relations therapies. The therapeutic implications of the different models are outlined in Table 9-1. Like the preceding models, object relations therapies use interpretation as a central element, but the focus is different. Instead of looking at Oedipal-phase conflicts based in drives, and in the defenses mobilized against them, object relations therapy pays attention to pre-Oedipal relations, particularly maternal ones. Where objects are incidental to one-person models, the internal object world is the primary target of investigation by therapists of the relational schools. Drive and ego psychologies presume that once the conflicts are resolved and/or the defenses improved, then relations will follow suit. Object relations psychologies maintain that correction of distorted object perceptions is the primary focus and that conflicts and symptoms will improve in due course.

(continues)

TABLE 9-1 | *Comparison of Therapy from the Major Perspectives*

	Drive	Ego	Object Relations	Self
Origin of pathology	Id impulses seek expression and gratification. Defenses mounted by ego and superego yield pathologic behavior and emotions.	Symptoms are produced by ego in a misplaced attempt at adaptation.	Symptoms reflect distorted object relations and/or attempts to substitute for them.	Symptoms are breakdown products of noncohesive self. Self-pathology is result of imbalance of mirroring and idealizing poles; a matter of deficit, not conflict.
Goals	- Real improvement in mental functioning - Acquisition of insight - Development of tolerance of drives - Ability to assess and accept oneself objectively - Freedom from tensions and inhibitions - Realignment of aggressive energies for self-preservation and achievement - Improved reality adjustment - Consistent and loyal interpersonal relations with well-chosen objects - Free function of abilities in productive work - Improved sublimation in recreation and avocation - Full heterosexual function	- Relief of affective symptoms - Conscious control over symptomatic behaviors - Recognition of defensive operations - Deliberate choice of defense mechanisms - Maturation of defenses to age-appropriate level - Improved interpersonal relations	- Perceptions of others grounded in reality - Conscious choices of objects based on current affective needs and ability of others to provide - Affective stability - Productive channeling of aggressive energies - Minimization of splitting (as defined by respective object relations theories)	- Removal of inhibitions to inherent push toward healthy development - Consistent self-identity - Selfobject needs appropriate to current maturity and environment - Affective stability - Capacity for self-soothing - Capacities for empathy, creativity, humor, wisdom, and acceptance of mortality

TABLE 9-1 | Comparison of Therapy from the Major Perspectives (continued)

	Drive	Ego	Object Relations	Self
Questions	- What drive urge is being expressed? - What unconscious ideas are forcing the drive wishes to be repressed? - What defenses is the ego using to deal with the urges? - How do the defenses themselves reflect the id's drives? - What compromise is ego maintaining among drive wish, defense, and reality?	- What defenses are operating against the drives? - How adaptive are they? - What affects are provoking them? - What tools of adaptation have failed to develop abnormally or at all? - What areas of the conflict-free sphere are inadequately developed? - What factors in the environment shaped the maladaptive or inadequate development of the ego?	- What is the nature of current object relations (as defined by respective object relations theories)? - At what developmental stage were object relations disrupted? - What injury, trauma, or deficit derailed normal object relations development? - What is the patient seeking from current relations?	- What is the nature of self-object needs? - What is the balance between mirroring and idealizing poles of development? - What injuries or deficiencies in the past prevented healthy development?
Nature and content of interventions	- Encouragement of free association and recollection of repressed ideas and emotions - Identification of id impulses and drive derivatives - Interpretation of conflicts that result in pathological phenomena	- Identification of affects - Identification of defense mechanisms at work - Elaboration of intended adaptive purpose of defenses	- Identification of distorted perceptions of and wishes from others - Identification of affective context of behaviors	- Identification of selfobject needs, particularly in transference - Effects of disruptions in selfobject matrix by failings of therapist

Continued

TABLE 9-1 Comparison of Therapy from the Major Perspectives (continued)

	Drive	Ego	Object Relations	Self
		- Identification of relevant life-stage issues in development - Assessment of adaptive value of perceptions and responses	- Identification of splitting of affects and/or objects - Clarification of consequences of relational distortions - Exploration of alternative perceptions and relations - Strong emphasis on object relations in transference - Countertransference is diagnostic of object relations pathology	- Healing effects of therapist's empathy - Specific avoidance of expectation of change
Transference	- Therapist is blank screen onto whom patient projects ongoing wishes, fears, and distortions - Analysis of transference is most productive realm for understanding drive impulses and defenses against them	- Therapist brings personal characteristics and behavior into the dyad; patient responds in attempts to adapt - Transference is most productive venue for understanding and changing patterns of maladaptive response	- Therapist is a specific individual who serves as the object of transference projections and brings his or her own character and behaviors into the dyad - Transference is inherently dyadic - Transference is necessary target of analysis and interpretation - Transference has curative potential (depending on specific object relations theory)	- Therapist is participant in selfobject matrix - Therapist is an individual who makes specific contributions to the transference dyad - Disruption by therapist's perceived failings is inevitable and serves a basis for disruption-restoration cycle of therapy

135

Since drive theory holds that pathology results from material that was improperly repressed, then cure requires that it be recovered, claimed, and appropriately internalized into the ego under conscious control. Object relations theory attributes pathology to wrongly internalized objects, and therefore successful therapy requires that those pathogenic objects be disowned and externalized in order to be replaced with more realistic ones.

Transference in drive and ego psychology is a projection of the patient's unconscious expectations onto the relatively neutral screen of the therapist. In the relational model, the patient still brings in his or her habitual patterns of perception, hope, and fear; but the therapist is no longer considered a blank slate. The transference instead is inherently dyadic. There are two very real human beings involved in a prolonged emotional encounter. The specifics of the therapist's appearance, demeanor, communication, and behavior all have particular reference in the patient's object world. The therapist is also affected, as the patient's emotions and projections influence his or her own feelings and fantasies. The object relations therapist is obliged to examine his or her particular responses to the patient, understand the contributions of his or her own unresolved issues, and assess what the patient has contributed to the interaction. Countertransference becomes not an impediment or complication, as it is in one-person psychologies, but an opportunity for emotionally based diagnostic scrutiny.

This perspective adds a dimension to the nature of interpretation. In the drive and ego models, interpretations convey information that uncovers unconscious motivations and brings them under conscious control of the ego. In the relational models, interpretation is also an interaction. Every communication from the therapist is conveyed in an affective context. Every action or intervention is an interpersonal event perceived through the template of the patient's mode of object relations. The patient is not only informed by an interpretation, he or she is also changed by the process of sharing it with the therapist. The therapist pays attention to the context of the interpretation, and to the patient's responses to it, and may use that observation as the focus of further interpretation.

Since pathology can all be traced to disturbed object relations, since those pathogenic patterns are predictably reenacted in the specific dyad of the transference, and since cure depends on correction of those relational distortions, it follows necessarily that the transference is a vehicle not only of diagnosis but also of therapy. To varying degrees, each of the object-relational schools views the therapeutic relationship as an opportunity for direct change in the maladaptive patterns of perception and response in which the patient's suffering is based. Through interpretation at least, and in some models by direct intervention, the therapist uses the transference as a corrective experience for the patient.

Guided by their respective models of normal human development and its vulnerabilities to maladjustment, the theories differ in other dimensions:

- The emphasis placed on the drives and their manifestations
- The focus on the self as an object of attention
- The degree of directive activity required of the therapist
- The degree to which the therapist attempts to become a corrective object in the patient's world

Each of the major object relations theorists owns a model of human development. Just as each model paints a different picture of how misdirected development produces pathological results, each points the therapist in a particular direction toward effecting change.

Melanie Klein

Klein's models pay particular attention to the object-based nature of the drives, to the primary role of fantasy in the object world, to the intensity of aggression as a driving force in normality and pathology, to the centrality of the conflict between love and hate, and to the persistence of the depressive position through adult life. In the domain of therapy, she dealt primarily with children and is perhaps best known for introducing play therapy as a technique. Her successors have adapted her models for psychotherapy with adults (mainly for psychoanalysis).

Kleinian therapy searches actively for the prevailing fantasies, since these elements are at the root of all relational experiences. Dreams, daydreams, and spontaneous elaborations are mined for their fantastic content. Stories of real-life events are reformulated around the presumptive fantasies at their center, as are reactions to the therapist. Presuming the presence of hidden aggressive impulses, and of love-hate conflicts, the therapist quite actively makes direct interpretations of the hypothesized meaning of the images in the fantasies. These explications often center on sadistic intentions and consequent guilt.

When MS. GRAY announced her desire to drive her car into a telephone pole, the therapist noted, "That seems like a very angry thing to do." Ms. Gray confirmed her anger and, with some facilitation by the therapist, she listed some of the many objects of her anger: Michael, her parents, her unpredictable moods. "And me?" queried the therapist. "I'm going to be leaving you in a few weeks. What are your ideas about that?" With that invitation, Ms. Gray elaborated her fantasies that the therapist was unable to tolerate Ms. Gray's emotions and that he was leaving her with Michael just as her mother had failed to protect her against her father. As she spoke, her hostility toward the therapist grew and she expressed her wish that his plane would crash on his vacation. When prompted for her feelings in the event that were actually to happen, she acknowledged she would feel avenged but terribly guilty. The therapist suggested that her own violent suicidal fantasy was an expression of self-punishment for her wish to kill the therapist.

While Freudian and ego-psychological therapists tend to avoid such intrusive interventions out of respect for the anxiety they could generate, Klein's model predicts that the patient's anxiety is lessened by such interventions. The reasoning is that anxiety results from fear of the power of the fantasies, and that the repression dictated by that fear produces even more symptoms. By making direct interpretations of the fantasies and the repressed drives they convey, the therapist provides a soothing demonstration that the psychic energies can be tolerated, and that the therapist is a reliable object, different from the feared ones in the patient's unconscious.

Such clarifications identify the split between idealized and persecutory object images and permit a more balanced perspective on contemporary relationships. They also allow for a reduction in depressive anxiety, as the power of the aggressive urges is lessened, the fear of harm to the object is framed more realistically, and the resultant guilt over hurt to the loved object is diminished. Hate is never eliminated, but it loses its infantile power to destroy love.

Margaret Mahler

Although Mahler's clinical work focused on patients with psychotic and severe personality disorders, and while her reflections on less severe disturbances of development were drawn from her observations of children, her followers have adapted her ideas in both realms to create a generalizable philosophy of therapy. As would be expected from her view of normal development, the focus is on deficits in separation and individuation. In fact, the phases of normal autism and normal symbiosis, as well as the differentiation and practicing subphases of the separation–individuation phase, are so primitive that one would be hard-pressed to imagine a candidate for depth psychotherapy who had not traversed these stages mostly successfully. Thus the primary foci of Mahlerian therapy are the subphases of rapprochement and libidinal object constancy.

In rapprochement, the tasks are to realize one's separateness from mother, to test reality, to contain infantile grandiosity, and to tolerate the inherent frustration of these achievements. The quality of affect is dictated by the quality of the object relationship. In treatment, the therapist notes residua of failures in these steps. Such failures might be manifest in idealization of the self or other and/or in impaired capacity to draw a clean line between self and other. Such imperfect connections are observed both in the stories the patient tells of his or her life outside therapy and in the transference.

MS. WHITE's therapist aimed to undo his patient's overinvestment in her children and her perception of her husband as encroaching on her space. He highlighted her tendency to idealize her children and to idealize her own centrality in their lives. In the context of the therapy, she was able to mobilize memories of her parents' reliable care for her and her fantasies of continuing that caring connection forever. "Caring for your children," prompted the therapist, "lets you believe that you'll never be left alone yourself." Ms. White agreed and associated to her expectation that her husband would do the same for her. Over time, she came to see that his postretirement presence in the home stood at odds with his former, almost mythic status as provider. With the therapist's encouragement, she gave voice to fantasies that his puttering in the home felt like his attempt to take away the support she wanted him to give. It seemed to her that he was wanting her to take care of him somehow. Looking at these constellations in the light of adult circumstances allowed her to acknowledge her wishes yet to disconnect them from contemporary expectations. The aim of the therapy going forward would be to foster a personal sense of individuality without resentment.

The therapist pays particular attention to split-off idealized and persecutory representations and recognizes the elements of the self and other in both. While Mahler had been among the first to note the necessity of a responsive real other ("the ordinarily de-voted mother" in the "average expectable environment"), she did not see that it was the task of therapy to replace directly deficits in these functions. While the therapist indeed has to provide an at-tuned environment, the curative process still comes primarily from insight. By clarifying the object distortions in the patient's perceptions, by identifying the elements of self and other in the undifferentiated clusters of hostile and affectionate affect, he or she provides the patient with the opportunity to make those dis-tinctions and to formulate more realistic object perceptions and re-sponses in the present. Since ego arises from the ability to await and expect satisfaction, the therapist's interventions nurture the development of these capacities in adult life, and thereby strengthen ego's mastery of affect and behavior.

W.R.D. Fairbairn

Fairbairn's contributions to the annals of therapy parallel his posi-tion among the theorists. He was an early radical, discarding both the id and the notion that drives inherently seek pleasure. Yet his ideas were so contrary to the mainstream of his own time that they found little foothold on their own and served mostly as stepping stones for later theorists. His approach to therapy was similarly sweeping, but because of the absence of a vital community putting it into practice and refining its ideas as an intellectual entity, it also served mostly as a way station for therapeutic evolution.

   Fairbairn's model of pathogenesis puts the blame for mis-guided development on a persisting split in the ego between rep-resentations of good and bad object experiences. The therapeutic necessity is to unify these ego elements. In limited writings, Fair-bairn saw insight into old and current object relationships as illus-trative and informative, but not curative. Healing instead requires the forging of real relationships with good objects that let the patient integrate the split-off representations of self and other. The only such relationship available in the therapy is that between patient and therapist. Thus the therapist provides the most trust-worthy environment possible, and both allows and encourages the patient to experience him or her as a good object. In doing so, he or she allows the patient to weaken the repression of bad objects and diminish the feared affects attached to them, allowing for fuller integration of the self.

D. W. Winnicott

Winnicott envisioned optimal development within a context of near-perfect attunement of mother and child. In his system, psychopathology results from a failure of this nurturing environment, necessitating the adoption of a false self. Friction between the true and false selves produces distress and symptoms.

His emphasis on the overwhelming influence of the environment extended to his view of the nature of psychotherapeutic cure. Regression is critical. First, regression in the therapy recreates the pathogenic constellation in the transference. It allows the therapist to see the point at which optimal development was derailed; when, where, and how the false self intervened. Therapeutic repair requires that development then be resumed at that point.

Such regression is permitted, and even fostered, by the analytic setting. The stable, soothing, reliable context of the therapy represents the holding environment. Within this safe situation, the patient can take the risk of letting go of the false self piece by piece. He or she experiences the therapist in his or her object world, as the early gratifying and/or frustrating mother. The therapist encourages expression of the true self which has previously been defensively withdrawn. While clarification and interpretation are as necessary as in other forms of psychodynamic therapy, here there is a specific expectation that the holding environment of the analysis is not just permissive of expression, but inherently curative. As the true self achieves expression, and as contradictory and conflicting object representations are consolidated, the healthy relationship with the therapist provides a contemporary environment within which derailed development can be successfully resumed.

Otto Kernberg

In Kernberg's developmental scheme, experiences are composed of basic relational units, comprising self-representation, object representation, and prevailing affect. Succession of such experiences, split into good and bad, gives rise to the libidinal and aggressive drives, respectively. The agency that represses bad experiences and retains the good is the ego, and the repressed experiences themselves constitute the id. Imbalances among the elements of such relational units can alter personality organization, and persistent pathology results when splits between good and bad, between libido and aggression, between fantasy and reality, between id and ego, cannot be accommodated or resolved. Kernberg focused most intensely on the borderline level of personality organization, marked by persistent splitting and affective instability.

Since affect and object representations are at the heart of both normal and unhealthy development, it stands to reason that those two elements stand at the core of Kernberg's model of therapy. It is in the transference that the assessment occurs. Patients may predictably describe situations outside the treatment setting, but the therapist listens for transference implications and makes most interpretations within the envelope of the transference dyad.

Technically, Kernberg and his followers pay particularly close attention to the predominant affect, and actively purse expression of emotion. The objective is not mere abreaction (i.e., feeling better by "getting it all out"), but specific identification of the affective dimension of the relational unit. The therapist deliberately elaborates the patient's perceptions of the therapist, perceptions of himself or herself, and feeling states.

MS. GRAY's sessions were always lively. The therapist came to expect Ms. Gray's cynical rejection of most of his interpretations. When she returned the week after he announced his vacation and informed him of her wish to die, he inquired about her mood. "I'm angry, of course," she replied. With little encouragement from him, she expanded on her anger at the therapist's unwillingness to help and at his selfish withholding of support. "If you're angry at me, why do you want to hurt yourself?" he asked with deliberate provocation. Ms. Gray was puzzled but intimated that she had trouble separating which emotions belonged to her and which belonged to others. The therapist confirmed his perception of that constellation and proposed that it was most comfortable to make the assignments so that the bad emotions always belonged to the other and the good ones to herself. By that schema, the therapist was selfish and inflexible, and Ms. Gray was kind and passive. She confirmed that the world did indeed seem that way to her. "But then," he continued, "when something threatens to tell you that maybe I can also do some good or that maybe you're being greedy, that's unacceptable, and you feel even worse." In the short run, Ms. Gray could understand and accept this formulation, but the therapist was certain it would require many future repetitions to effect lasting change.

Where earlier theorists used such transference interactions mostly as demonstrations of the patient's recurring needs and vulnerabilities, Kernberg also used it to identify projected images. Negative perceptions of the therapist are conceived to be projective identifications, i.e., representations of the self that cannot be tolerated within the ego and which must be unconsciously attributed to the therapist. Since it is precisely the suppression of these ideas and feelings which generates pathogenic conflict, it is incumbent on the therapist to mobilize and identify them vigorously. Simultaneously, he or she identifies the reciprocal (usually good) representations which are split off and retained within the patient's self representation.

Expectedly, such clarifications are initially met with denial and emotional chaos. The therapist identifies this resistance as the patient's reaction to the split emotions and ideas. With repeated encounters, the patient comes to identify repressed parts of himself or herself in those representations projected onto the therapist. The therapy proceeds with attempts to recall the origins of these distortions and splits and the circumstances that bred them. With repeated interpretation, the patient's ego is able to reabsorb and integrate those aspects that were tossed out and thereby to lessen the intensity of conflict among and between drives and structures. The aim is to expand partial representations of objects into more complete ones and to allow primitive transferences to develop into more mature ones.

SELF PSYCHOLOGY

Self psychology rejects the drives and structures that form the foundations of the other theories. The core concept is that of the self, an overarching function that ties together all of an individual's experiences, perceptions, and identity. Normally, selfobject experiences provide sources of both mirroring and idealization, allowing for the development of a balanced self with strong cohesion. Faulty selfobject experiences at critical developmental phases produce particular imbalances between the poles of the bipolar self with pathological manifestations particular to the selfobject experience and the developmental phase. Quite vigorously, self psychology maintains that all psychopathology is the result of deficit, not conflict, and that the symptoms that bring people to therapy are the breakdown products of a self whose cohesion is threatened.

Since this weak self is at the center of all pathology, it must follow that the object of therapy is to strengthen the self. Some of the aims of earlier models, such as bringing the unconscious to conscious awareness, resolving conflicting ideas and emotions, and remembering repressed experiences, may be tools for the task of fortifying the self, and they are almost sure to follow as capacities of the strengthened self; but they are not themselves the aims of the therapy.

This formulation presents an obvious problem: If the self is enfeebled by injurious past experiences, how can the therapy provide a cure? Indeed, it is a common and erroneous criticism of self psychology that it attempts to cure past experiences by substituting better ones in the present. In fact, one cannot undo the past, and the self psychologist does not aim to do so. Instead, he or she allows the thwarted path of natural development to unfold in a healthy way by re-experiencing old situations in a new context. The instinct for development is built in. The therapist and patient create situations that allow it to resume. Indeed, the literature of this model often uses the term "restoration" to identify the curative process experienced by the self in therapy.

Essential to the process, as it is in all forms of psychodynamic therapy, is a setting that encourages self expression. Two ingredients are vital:

- The therapist's *empathy* stands at the core of the entire curative process and is critical to the entire therapeutic environment. Particularly, empathy means seeing the patient's situation from his or her perspective. The therapist must make constant and consistent efforts to avoid confusing empathy with *sympathy*, i.e., putting himself or herself into the patient's situation and imagining his or her own reactions, or feeling pity for the patient's circumstances. Empathy in this context has been described as "temporary indwelling" or "vicarious introspection." It requires the therapist to imagine himself or herself behind the patient's eyes and in the patient's shoes, while retaining his or her own objectivity and perspective.
- Simultaneously, the therapist must be *nonjudgmental*. Whatever the patient describes about himself or herself, or about others in the past or present environment, the therapist retains the presumption that this person is not bad but human. To judge the patient negatively is to put him or her

in jeopardy in the transference; to judge the patient positively only makes it likely that a negative judgment is forthcoming in the near future. To judge others, even as the
patient does, is to substitute sympathy for empathy and
similarly to threaten the safety of the therapeutic setting.

The Disruption–Restoration Process

In such a setting, therapeutic regression naturally takes place.
From the perspective of this psychology, regression means the
reawakening of archaic selfobject relations. The selfobject experiences that are revived in the transference, of course, will reflect all
the deficits that bring the patient to therapy in the first place.
Within the empathic and nonjudgmental context of the therapy,
those selfobject needs become more fluid and changeable.

The point behind the elaboration of these primitive selfobject
experiences is to replace them with needs and perceptions that
are more appropriate to the contemporary setting. The therapist
expects that the patient has more cognitive and behavioral options than he or she did in the original environment and can use
those resources to alter the nature of his or her selfobject needs.
Since the maturation of these selfobject experiences is the aim of
therapy and since they are only accessible through the transference, it is axiomatic that true restoration of the healthy self
occurs only in and through the transference. A technical dictate
of self-psychological theory is that the therapist should never in-
terfere with the development of the selfobject transference.

But, just as they did with Sigmund Freud, patients will resist
the expression of selfobject experiences in the transference. In self
psychology, this resistance is seen not as a complication, but as an
expected phenomenon and as an opportunity. The patient's resistance to the transference is a fear of being injured, traumatized, or
disappointed, as was his or her experience in the past. Understanding of the transference begins with understanding of the
resistance to it. In identifying the inherent fears, patient and
therapist come to a first level of understanding of the selfobject
experience. By knowing what disappointment or rejection the
patient fears, the therapist understands the underlying needs.

Just as resistance is seen as an opportunity rather than an impediment, so, too, are the therapist's failures viewed as openings for
understanding and intervention. The self-psychological therapist

does not provide a corrective emotional experience to replace the harmful ones in the patient's past. Since he or she is human, he or she will necessarily disappoint some element of the patient's selfobject needs. Instead, such junctures are a piece of process that alternates between disruption and restoration. Selfobject needs are mobilized in the regressed transference. Fears from the past are also carried along and serve to protect against repeated injury. When the therapist provides an incompletely empathic interpretation; when he or she fails to live up to the patient's desire for constant and immediate availability; when any of the therapist's human failings resonate with an archaic need or fear, the selfobject matrix is disrupted. The patient often becomes symptomatic in a manner consistent with the patterns that brought him or her to therapy. The therapist notes and interprets the disruption and places it in context of the patient's wishes and fears. The result is not only repair of the damage to the matrix but growth in the strength of the self.

MS. WHITE told the therapist about her weekly bridge game the previous evening. One of her friends, Elaine, made a comment about Ms. White's hair that the patient took to be demeaning, although to the therapist it sounded fairly neutral. Ms. White felt uneasy for the rest of the card game and continued to ruminate about the slight. The therapist offered the possibility that what Elaine had said reflected negative judgments Ms. White held about herself. Ms. White replied, "Yes, that may be true," and then lapsed into an unaccustomed silence. After a few minutes, the therapist asked what Ms. White was feeling, and she gave a benign and nonspecific reply. He followed with, "How did you feel after I speculated about your reaction to Elaine's comment?"

"I felt sort of embarrassed, like I should have known that, and it was silly for me to have those sorts of feelings about myself and about Elaine." The therapist then reflected that it hurt to have him point out to her that she was being silly and immature. Ms. White was able to elaborate that indeed she felt sad about his comment. Looking deeper, therapist and patient found that she wished for the therapist to respect her, not to look down on her.

Hearing a manifestation of a frustrated need for mirroring, the therapist returned with Ms. White to the events of the card game. Ms. White reflected that she admired Elaine's sense of style and always got a lift out of her infrequent compliments. The therapist corrected his earlier interpretation and offered, "It sounds as if you were sad that Elaine didn't give you a compliment after you had put effort into doing your hair, and her comment hurt you." Ms. White acknowledged that

> such a reading felt more correct than the first one and expanded on the affective details of the event.
>
> The therapist was then able to point out how his first interpretation, which was indeed off the mark, left her feeling hurt and sad in the same way as Elaine's comment the night before. After a few moments' reflection, Ms. White confirmed how much she wished for the therapist to admire and compliment her and how frightened she often was to describe her foibles to him. She elaborated with an early memory of how enlivened she felt when her father complimented her looks before a date in her youth.

Notably, self psychology mandates that interpretations of such disruptions clarify the role of the therapist, the behavior, or the communication that stimulated the disruption of the selfobject matrix. Healing is the outcome of both being understood by the other and having an effect on the other. With each successive episode of transference frustration followed by corrective interpretation, the patient becomes less of a victim and more of a partner. The archaic selfobject relationship with the therapist is, bit by bit, supplanted by a more mature, reciprocal, collaborative one. This experience of efficacy is a vital ingredient of the therapeutic process that fortifies the patient's self.

This cycle in self-psychological treatment is often framed as the "disruption–restoration" process. The patient enters therapy with archaic selfobject needs, which are evoked anew in the therapeutic setting. Inevitably, the needs are perceived to be frustrated and some disruption of the therapist–patient relationship ensues. Effective analysis of the disruption not only sheds light on transference distortions, it also provides a building block for a more adaptive level of selfobject relations. Steps in the process are:

- Resistance analysis—It is natural for patients to resist expressions of their archaic wishes, not simply out of embarrassment, but also out of fear that those wishes will again be frustrated. The analyst, sensitive to manifestations of those wishes, points out the resistances. That act in itself helps to overcome the fear of frustration that underlies the resistance in the first place.
- Transference mobilization—Since transference is ubiquitous, it is always ready to emerge. Repeated analysis of resistance and continual demonstrations of empathic

sensitivity facilitate the emergence of the selfobject transference at the patient's psychological core.

■ Transference disruption—The therapist, simply a human
being, must fall short of transference expectations from
time to time. Taking a vacation when the patient is facing a
stressful event or offering an interpretation that is "out of
tune" in the patient's ears are but two common ways the
therapist may contribute to disruption of the transference.
One technical implication of the philosophy behind self
psychology is that the therapist first acknowledges the
reality of the event that precipitated the disruption, making
the patient's reaction understandable and thus providing
leverage for a mutative interpretation.

■ Transference regression—In virtually all the schools of
thought examined in this volume, contemporary stressors
or frustrations can precipitate regression to a less mature
stage of perception or thought. Here, too, frustration of the
selfobject needs in the therapy yields a regression in the
transference. Temporarily, the patient manifests more archaic selfobject desires and modes of interaction. In the face
of a threat to a particular selfobject constellation, the patient defensively reverts to a more primitive form to protect
the remaining self structure. Analysis of such regressions
exposes the most basic selfobject needs and contributes a
linear, developmental perspective to the analytic portrayal
of the patient's selfobject world.

■ Restoration—Interpretation of the basic needs and the
emotional effect of their frustration puts the mature elements of the patient's self in alliance with the therapist as
examiners and fixers of the weaknesses of the self. It is only
through the necessary disruptions of the selfobject matrix
that the opportunity exists for this new selfobject experience to be forged. An essential ingredient of this new relationship is that it propels the patient toward autonomy
without a sense of abandonment or betrayal.

Mutative Interpretation

In order for an intervention to be mutative (i.e., to make a lasting
change in the patient's self), it must:

■ evoke an emotional experience;
■ involve the transference, and

include understanding of the contributions of both the patient and the therapist, with no blame on either.

Emotion is the energetic force behind both pathology and cure, so mutative interventions must center on emotional experiences, not simply intellectual ones. And, since the live emotions in the therapist's office are concurrent with the analytic process, they have a valence not achievable with tales of outside events and relationships. Human failings and the resultant disturbance of the transference matrix provide the prime opportunities for such mutative interventions. Repeated encounters of that sort facilitate the patient's abilities to accept imperfections in himself or herself and others.

It is a controversial tenet of self psychology that the therapist does not expect the patient to change. He or she may often see how the patient might suffer less by thinking, acting, or communicating differently, but that is not the aim of the therapy. Instead, it is viewed as an opportunity for the patient to acquire the needed stability and strength that have been deficient in previous development and to remove the impediments to the patient's natural urge to get healthy. Indeed, the demand for change may have been part of the early selfobject failings that interfered with development of the cohesive self. In therapy, if change occurs, it is the consequence of psychic growth.

It is necessary, but not sufficient, for interpretations to be correct. An interpretation that explains behavior, thought, or feeling in a way that is new and instructive does not by itself produce change. Rather, it is the therapist's ability to understand the patient empathically, to provide respect and real contact that is curative. The self can only grow within a selfobject matrix. Correct interpretations allow the transference matrix to persist, but it is the human interaction that changes the patient's self.

Critics have argued that self psychology suffers from its failure to be more demanding of patients and counts on the patient to be cured by the kindness and empathy of the therapist. Ernest Wolf (1999, p. 117) has countered, "Neither empathy nor love cures." Therapeutic empathy includes both understanding and explaining. It provides rational, verbal expression to the meaning of behavior and emotion. Empathy often illuminates the necessity of frustration in order for the patient to grow from the process of disruption and restoration. The therapist's attitudes provide a matrix in which the patient's self can become embedded and resume its natural progress toward health.

Learning points

- Object relations models (especially those of Fairbairn, Winnicott, and Kernberg), as well as self psychology, use the transference relationship not only as the most accurate diagnostic window to the patient's problems, but also as a direct instrument of therapy.
- In all relational models, the affective context and content of experiences is a central focus.
- In all these models, the context of delivering an interpretation is at least as important as the content of the interpretation.
- Object relations theories identify splitting (as defined by the respective models) and aim to rectify pathogenic splitting through the therapy.
- Self psychology emphasizes the importance of empathy as both a diagnostic tool and an instrument of healing.
- Self psychology anticipates disruptions in the selfobject matrix of the transference and uses restoration of the matrix as a central element of therapeutic change.

RECOMMENDED READINGS

Kernberg O. *Object-Relations Theory and Clinical Psychoanalysis*. New York: Jason Aronson, 1976.

Kohut H. *How Does Analysis Cure?* Chicago: University of Chicago Press, 1984.

Masterson JF, Tolpin M, Sifneos PE. *Comparing Psychoanalytic Psychotherapies: Developmental, Self, and Object Relations: Self Psychology, Short-Term Dynamic*. New York: Brunner/Mazel, 1991.

Scharff Jill S, Scharff David E. *Object Relations Individual Therapy*. Northvale, NJ: Jason Aronson, 1998.

Winnicott DW. *Holding and Interpretation*. New York: Grove Press, 1987.

Wolf ES. *Treating the Self: Elements of Clinical Self Psychology*. New York: Guilford Press, 1988.

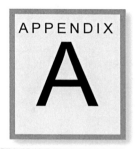

APPENDIX

A

Glossary of Psychodynamic Terminology

adaptation–the process of coping with the environment in order to optimize physical and emotional survival. Adaptation may be alloplastic (changing the environment) or autoplastic (changing some part of the self). Heinz Hartmann saw adaptation as the driving force behind ego development.

archetype–an inborn tendency to sense things in a certain way, organized around stereotypes. In Carl Jung's model, archetypes include such figures as mother and hero. The collective unconscious is organized around these archetypes.

collective unconscious–an inborn collection of potentials that all humans share. Central to Jung's model, the collective unconscious is inherited across cultures and constitutes the transpersonal element of the human psyche.

conflict–struggle among, between, or within psychic structures or between structures and reality. In drive, ego, and object relations psychologies, conflict propels both normal development and psychopathology.

conflict-free sphere–the realm of development that proceeds of its own energy. In Hartmann's developmental scheme, this sphere includes such functions as locomotion, perception, and memory.

defense–ego's attempt to protect against, or cope with, threats. Defense mechanisms are the specific methods employed by the ego to cope with internal or external threats. (See Table 3-1.)

depressive position–an object relations configuration that accepts the good and bad aspects of objects, but still believes in the destructive power of aggressive impulses. In Melanie Klein's scheme, the child in this position is fearful of the effects of his or her hostile wishes on the object of libidinal attachment. This position begins in about the fourth month and continues throughout life.

151

drive–a motivational force that impels human behavior. In Sigmund Freud's model, the two drives are aggression and libido.

ego–the psychic structure that manages the demands of id, superego, and reality. The ego mounts the defense mechanisms and contains the object world. It also develops and implements capacities including locomotion, memory, and speech.

empathy–the capacity to share the perspective and experience of another person. In self psychology, this function of "vicarious introspection" is necessary for normal development and for effective psychotherapy.

epigenetic model–the scheme elaborated by Erik Erikson to describe the succession of tasks and crises faced by the ego in a lifelong process of development.

false self–a configuration of attitudes and behaviors adopted in reaction to the demands of objects who cannot appreciate and respond to one's genuine innate potentials. In D.W. Winnicott's model of object relations, the struggle between the true and false selves is at the core of psychopathology.

fragmentation–loss of cohesion of the self, usually under stress. In self psychology, pathological symptoms are manifestations of fragmentation, the breakdown products of deficient self-cohesion.

holding environment–the state in which the caregiver, usually the mother, anticipates and provides the child's needs and protects him or her from discomfort. D.W. Winnicott saw this environment as the breeding ground for the healthy ego and as a necessity for adaptive object relations.

id–the structure that contains the mental representations of the drives. In Sigmund Freud's structural model, id is innate; ego and superego arise from it. In Heinz Hartmann's ego psychological model, id and ego arise from an undifferentiated matrix; in Otto Kernberg's object relations model, id is the product of material repressed by ego.

inferiority complex–a pervasive feeling of lacking in many qualities or of being substantially imperfect. In Alfred Adler's model, the inferiority complex lies at the base of many neurotic emotions and behaviors.

interpersonal psychoanalysis–a diverse school of thought unified by an underlying premise that human thinking, emotion, and behavior reflected the influence of the social environment. Its chief proponents were Harry Stack Sullivan, Karen Horney, and Erich Fromm.

interpretation–the process of putting into words the therapist's understanding of a patient's mental life. Interpretations may explain the nature of a current mental process and/or its source.

latent content–the underlying intent of a dream. Sigmund Freud assumed that latent content was always representative of wish fulfillment.

manifest content–the story and images perceived by the dreamer. Latent content is converted to manifest content by the process of dream work.

mirroring–the confirmation by a selfobject of one's goodness and wholeness. In self psychology, mirroring selfobjects promote the development of the pole of self-assertive ambitions.

neurosis–a complex of psychiatric symptoms resulting from intrapsychic conflict. Sigmund Freud termed these conditions "psychoneuroses" to differentiate them from "actual neuroses," which are no longer given any credence. In most nosologic schemes, reality testing is intact in neuroses, differentiating them from psychoses.

Oedipal crisis (or Oedipus complex)–a constellation of desires and ideas involving a wish for union with the opposite-sex parent and destruction of the same-sex parent. Drive psychology considers these desires fairly literally, while ego psychology and object relations theories treat them more or less metaphorically. The Oedipal crisis usually occurs around ages 3 through 6; the Oedipus complex is its adult residue.

optimal frustration–a nontraumatic failure to gratify a person's needs. In self psychology, it is a necessary element that fosters new learning and personal growth, both in normal development and in psychotherapy.

paranoid position–a primitive object relations configuration in which hostile impulses are projected onto objects. In Melanie Klein's scheme, this position characterizes the first 3 months of life and is accompanied by the fear of abandonment or destruction by bad objects.

parapraxis–an error of everyday life that reflects repressed unconscious motives. Such an error is commonly called a "Freudian slip."

preconscious–the system of mental content not within conscious awareness, but available for retrieval with effort. Most nonrepressed memory is in the preconscious.

primary process–the earliest, most primitive form of mental function. It is directly connected to drive impulses and seeks immediate discharge. Primary process uses symbols and substitutions freely and has no regard for chronology. It is characteristic of unconscious mental operations and shapes the manifest content of dreams.

psychic determinism–one of the central hypotheses of psychoanalysis, which maintains that all psychic activity and behavior has meaning, and derives from psychic events that came before.

secondary process–the mature form of mental function. Characteristic of conscious mental activity, it uses verbal representation and readily understood symbols. It respects the order of time and avoids contradictions and inconsistencies.

secondary revision–the process of changing dream content after waking. Secondary revision can be both conscious and unconscious and can be presumed to influence all dreams reported in therapy.

selfobject–the subjective experience of another person or entity. In self psychology, it is more properly termed the selfobject experience and occurs within a shared selfobject matrix.

separation–individuation–in Margaret Mahler's formulation, the major process of development of autonomy and identity. Separation is the differentiation of self from other, and individuation is the process of defining the self. This process begins at about age 5 months, and continues throughout life.

signal anxiety–tension that arises in the anticipation of a dangerous development or traumatic occurrence. In Sigmund Freud's formulation, signal anxiety triggers defense mechanisms that prevent the emergence of overwhelming affect, but may also lead to neurotic levels of distress.

splitting–the process of separating psychological content by extremes or opposites. In the object relations school, splitting is defined by various theorists between good and bad objects, between affect and cognition, and between self and object. Splitting is a primitive mental process that usually yields pathological results in adult life.

structural model–the system of id, ego, and superego. Sigmund Freud defined the structural model (also called the "tripartite model") in 1923.

superego–the mental structure that contains ideals and prohibitions. In Sigmund Freud's model, it is a product of the Oedipal crisis.

topographic model–the system of unconscious, preconscious, and conscious. It was Sigmund Freud's first model of mental operations, articulated in 1915.

transitional object–an inanimate object invested by the child with magical properties of soothing and comfort. In D.W. Winncott's model, it is the first product of the child's creativity.

unconscious–that system of mental operations entirely outside awareness. In Sigmund Freud's topographic model, it is evident only through the effort of free association or through its manifestation in dreams, parapraxes, and symptoms.

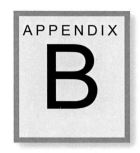

APPENDIX

B

Chronology of Major Contributors to Psychodynamic Theory

Drive	1840	1860	1880	1900	1920	1940	1960	1980	2000

Josef Breuer (1842–1925)
Freud's first collaborator

Sigmund Freud (1856 –1939)
Founder of psychoanalysis

Alfred Adler (1870–1937)
Inferiority complex

Carl Jung (1875–1961)
Collective unconscious; archetypes

Karl Abraham (1877–1925)
Oral, anal, phallic characters

Ernest Jones (1879–1958)
Translation of Freud into English

Otto Rank (1884–1939)
Birth trauma; psychology of art and society

(continues)

Ego

1840	1860	1880	1900	1920	1940	1960	1980	2000	

Anna Freud (1895–1982)
Ego mechanisms of defense

Heinz Hartmann (1894–1970)
Adaptive functions of ego

Franz Alexander (1891–1964)
Psychosomatic medicine; brief psychotherapy

Erik Erikson (1902–1994)
Epigenetic model of development

George Vaillant (1934–)
Maturation of defenses

Interpersonal

Harry Stack Sullivan (1892–1949)
Interpersonal psychoanalysis

Karen Horney (1885–1952)
Interpersonal dimensions of neurosis

Erich Fromm (1900–1980)
Social-historical context

John Bowlby (1907–1990)
Attachment theory

(continues)

	1840	1860	1880	1900	1920	1940	1960	1980	2000

Object relations

Melanie Klein (1882–1960)
Fantasy and aggression

Margaret Mahler (1897–1985)
Separation–individuation

W.R.D. Fairbairn (1889–1964)
Object-seeking libido

D.W. Winnicott (1896–1971)
True and false selves

Edith Jacobson (1897–1978)
Self representation in object world; affective tension

Otto Kernberg (1928–)
Primacy of affect and splitting

Self

Heinz Kohut (1913–1981)
Founder of self psychology

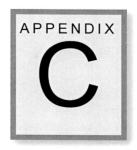

APPENDIX

C

An Outline for Comprehensive Psychodynamic Formulation

ANDREW B. KLAFTER

INTRODUCTION

A *psychodynamic formulation* is an explanation of how a patient's psychological development and personal history have led to his or her symptoms and problems, pattern of interpersonal relationships, cognitive style, affective responses, and impulse regulation. A psychodynamic formulation should immediately suggest how a therapeutic relationship with the psychotherapist will lead to symptom relief or foster growth and change, and should provide direction toward specific foci and techniques for successful psychotherapy treatment.

The following system was developed at the University of Cincinnati Psychiatry Residency Training Program. It was originally developed as an outline and worksheet to help psychiatric residents apply the psychodynamic concepts they learn in didactic seminars to their clinical experiences. It is applicable, however, for any psychodynamic psychotherapists, including social workers or clinical psychologists. Students of psychotherapy are typically exposed to various psychodynamic concepts from their supervisors, readings, and didactic lectures. Often, they learn about concepts which originate in different psychoanalytic schools of thought. There is a widespread sentiment among many psychotherapy educators that it is healthy for residents to be exposed to a diversity of psychodynamic thinking. At the same time, however, consistency and clarity are essential in order to successfully impart the fundamental concepts of any field of knowledge, including psychodynamic psychotherapy and psychoanalysis. Without an understanding of how each of the major psychoanalytic approaches (drive theory, ego psychology, object relations, and self psychology) conceptualizes personality development and the psychotherapeutic process, it can be quite confusing when each supervisor or instructor conceptualizes the same clinical phenomena differently.

An example from my own training is illustrative: When one supervisor gave guidance about making interpretations, he intended for me to help my patient become more aware of her unconscious wishes and feelings. A second supervisor strongly disapproved of "id-interpretations" and instead encouraged me only to "convey empathy" in order to establish myself as a "positive object" so the patient could experience herself in a new, less critical light. I now realize that these supervisors formulate their cases according to different psychoanalytic ideas, and that the suggestions of each therapist made perfect sense from the point of view of how he understood my patient's problems. At the time, however, this experience furthered a caricature of psychoanalytic thinking as sloppy, self-contradictory, and incomprehensible.

In the present text, Dr. Bienenfeld addresses these challenges by offering the reader a general and broad introduction to each of the major schools of psychoanalytic thinking (drive theory, ego psychology, object relations, and self psychology) prior to delineating the salient theories, concepts, and techniques of each approach. Showing how each psychoanalytic concept comes from a particular school of thought provides important context. This approach is also helpful when formulating psychotherapy cases.

JARGON AND TECHNICAL LANGUAGE

One common misconception by novice psychotherapists about formulations is that they ought to be shrouded in technical jargon. To the contrary, a psychodynamic formulation should make things clearer, and not more mysterious. Psychodynamic psychotherapists often use technical terms ("Oedipus complex," "primitive-defenses," "selfobject," etc.) because they serve as shorthand for complex and widely accepted psychoanalytic ideas which would be very difficult to explain concisely with lay language. One word or phrase encapsulates ideas which might take an entire paragraph to describe. However, it is a very useful exercise for psychiatric residents (as well as their supervisors!) to avoid, whenever possible, using technical jargon. In fact, this exercise is formally implemented by some psychotherapy educators because the act of repeatedly explaining complex ideas in ordinary language helps us refine our understanding.

BIOLOGY AND SOCIAL ENVIRONMENT

Psychodynamic psychotherapy and psychoanalysis are not naïve to the impact of genetics and biology in psychological development. In addition, many patients are confronted with real-life problems (poverty, overwhelming dependent-care responsibilities, lack of transportation) which need to be dealt with practically because of their direct impact on patients' lives or their interference with the ability of patients to participate in psychotherapy treatment. (In many cases, it may not appropriate for the therapist to be the person who makes such interventions directly; rather, the therapist would point the patient in the direction of social services, an attorney, etc.) Therefore, a psychodynamic formulation is the psychological component of a comprehensive Bio-Psycho-Social understanding of a patient's problems. It would be irresponsible for a psychodynamic psychotherapist, when evaluating a patient with symptoms of depression, to ignore the fact that numerous relatives of the patient have had severe mood disorders which appear to have responded well to medications. Similarly, if a patient is confronted with formidable life problems, the formulation must seriously consider the impact of these issues.

USING THIS OUTLINE

The following outline and worksheet are intended to be used by psychotherapy trainees as an exercise which will guide them through a comprehensive consideration of the biological, psychodynamic, and social environmental factors which should be considered when evaluating psychotherapy patients for treatment. This format assumes that the treatment provider doing the assessment and formulation is a psychiatrist, and is licensed to prescribe medication as well as provide psychotherapy. However, this worksheet is easily applied to nonphysician therapists who are providing treatment in collaboration with a psychopharmacologist.

This outline is intended to be self-explanatory, but the psychiatric residents at University of Cincinnati who have worked with the worksheet have been able to make better use of it after first seeing it implemented by faculty members. In our training program, an eight-week seminar on psychodynamic formulation has been introduced, during which the instructor presents a psychotherapy case. Residents participating in the seminar are guided through the worksheet and formulate the case as a group. Applying psychodynamic ideas to a living case provides many opportunities for useful discussions about how human personality develops and how psychotherapy works. By the end of the seminar, residents are asked to present clinical vignettes and to formulate their own cases independently.

This written format attempts to simulate the manner in which psychotherapy cases are presented to supervisors or seminars. The outline and worksheet are included, first, in blank form so that they can be copied for use by readers who wish to follow this system for their own case formulations. A psychodynamic psychotherapy case is described in detail. The case is then formulated according to psychodynamic ideas. The patient's dynamics are briefly discussed, highlighting some important concepts which are well illustrated by this case. Then, the outline is applied to the psychotherapy case, and the reader has an opportunity to see how the worksheet can be used as an exercise to consider, comprehensively, various aspects of a patient's life history and current functioning.

The novel aspects of this outline are the worksheets which assist describing each case from the perspectives of drives and ego psychology, object relations, and self psychology. Drive theory and ego psychology have been merged into one section of the worksheet. This reflects my opinion that unconscious wishes are better understood when there is careful attention to the mechanisms of defense which modulate how these drives impact the patient's feelings, thoughts, and behavior. The worksheet on object relations is kept deliberately generic so that the ideas of any of the major object relations theorists would be applicable. What is most important for students of psychotherapy to note when evaluating patients from an object relations perspective is whether or not one can identify a pattern of relationships, or a "recurring drama," in which a patient finds himself or herself repeatedly entangled over time. The self psychology section is designed to be flexible in order to accommodate the virtually limitless ways that patients feel about themselves. Students who are familiar with the technical terms for selfobject transferences (mirroring, idealizing, twinship/alter-ego, etc.) are free to use these terms. What is probably more useful, however, is a simple description in ordinary terms of how important people in a patient's life have influenced that patient's view of himself or herself.

CHOOSING ONE PERSPECTIVE OR WORKING WITH MANY

Many therapists operate with a multiplicity of perspectives at the same time. For a given patient, one can ask the following questions. "What unconscious wishes and defenses are causing my patient to keep forgetting her mother's birthday?" "Why is it that the patient is attributing to me a very critical attitude which is very reminiscent of how her father has treated her?" Or, "How did this patient's negative review by her boss cause her to feel about herself, and can this help us understand why she slashed her co-worker's tires?" All of these might be useful questions for the same patient. Over the course of a psychotherapist's career, he or she may tend to use one perspective more than the others when understanding his or her patient's difficulties. Alternatively, some therapists find one model more helpful for one type of patient and another model better for a different group of patients. When starting off as a therapist, one has not yet had enough experiences to form a bias. Novice therapists are probably influenced by the perspectives of their supervisors as well as their own intuitive sense of how compelling they find each theory that they learn about. One of the purposes of this worksheet exercise is to give psychotherapy trainees an opportunity to attempt to formulate each patient from *all* the major psychoanalytic perspectives, and to then see for themselves how successful each model is in suggesting how psychotherapy treatment might be helpful. Therefore, it is expected that for a given case, one or the other model will be easier to apply. However, it is important to consider all of them before settling on one.

Outline and Worksheet for Bio-Psycho-Social Psychotherapy Case Formulation

*Patient:*_____   *Date:*_____

*Therapist:*_____

1. BIOLOGICAL FACTORS

a. Family psychiatric history and genetic vulnerability to psychiatric conditions:

b. Birth and developmental history, head injuries, other neurological problems, past and current medical conditions, and their impact on psychiatric illness and symptoms:

c. Current medications and their impact on psychiatric illness and symptoms:

d. Substance use/misuse and its impact on psychiatric illness and symptoms:

2. SOCIAL FACTORS

a. Financial situation (monthly income, source of income, monthly expenses):

b. Employment (job stability, relationship with boss/coworkers, work-related stress or other problems):

c. Supportive relationships (or lack thereof/social isolation) (Are friends, family, or neighbors available to help patient with errands, child care, etc?):

d. Recent disruption of relationships (break-ups, divorce, people who have moved out of town and how is patient coping):

e. Other recent losses/grief:

f. Legal problems:

g. Crises in lives of important people in patient's life (health, financial, or legal problems in relatives/partner/friends):

h. Access to medical and psychiatric care, affordability of proposed treatment:

3. PSYCHOLOGICAL FACTORS
   a. Drives and ego functions (see worksheet at end of outline)

   b. Object relations (see worksheet at end of outline)

   c. Self psychology (see worksheet at end of outline)

4. PROPOSED TREATMENT:
   a. Medications (category, agent, dose, goals for symptom improvement, and method/plan for monitoring symptoms):

   b. Social interventions (connection with social service agencies, notification of Child Protective Services, or Adult Protective Services, etc.):

   c. Psychotherapy
      i. Modality of therapy:

      ii. Length of treatment (open-ended vs. time-limited, number of sessions anticipated):

iii. Issues of focus (related to above issues in the formulation):

iv. Current or anticipated transferences and
    countertransferences:

d. Consultations with other professionals (M.D. for medication
   evaluation, psychologist for neuropsychological testing,
   primary care physician or medical/surgical specialist for
   evaluation/treatment):

a. Drives and Ego Functions

Symptoms, negative feelings, reported difficulties, other problems	Defenses and coping mechanisms	Underlying or disavowed wishes, drives, or beliefs against which the defenses are directed	Superego admonitions against disavowed wishes	How successful are these defenses or coping mechanisms? How aware is patient of underlying wishes? Is reality testing preserved? How are these defenses helpful or adaptive? What problems do they cause?

(continues)

168

b. Object Relations (Impact of Relationships on Internal Mental Life)

Objects (parents or caregiver, siblings, spouse, peers, boss, mentors, or other important persons in the patient's life)	Characterize this relationship over time. Describe the success or lack thereof of early and sustained *attachment* to this object, *unmet needs, ungratified wishes, conflicts,* and struggles.	Does this relationship fall into a *typical pattern or theme* which is comparable with the other relationships listed?	Does the patient's <u>transference</u> to the psychotherapist resemble this relationship? How does the therapist respond (*countertransference or enactments*) to the patient's transference?

(continues)

c. Self Psychology

Self-representations: (Included are common examples of important self-representations. Other terms may be more relevant for a specific patient)	Selfobjects (Identify important people, activities, possessions, etc., that influence the patient's self-representations)	Selfobject transferences (i.e., how does this selfobject influence the patient's self-representations? E.g., mirroring, idealizing, twining)	Defensive and compensatory mechanisms (i.e., what does the patient do in response to these self-representations and the emotional impact of these self-objects—is this response adaptive, maladaptive?)
safe, stable, powerful or *threatened, assaulted, impotent*			
attractive, well liked, lovable, loved or *unattractive, unpopular, rejected, unloved*			
intelligent, competent, effective, significant or *unintelligent, incompetent, insignificant, or worthless*			

IN-DEPTH CASE PRESENTATION

Initial Presentation

Miss R. is a 25-year-old female, who was a Ph.D. candidate in mathematics at the time of her initial presentation. She presented with most symptoms of major depression, including hypersomnia, fatigue, poor concentration, depressed mood, anhedonia, and reduced libido. She was unable to work more than 2 to 3 hours per day on her research and was afraid she'd be thrown out of the doctoral program. She diagnosed herself with "Chronic Fatigue Syndrome" (CFS). At the opening of the initial evaluation, she stated, "Before I give you any more information, I need to know whether you believe in CFS." The psychiatrist responded, "I don't know much about CFS, but I do believe that it exists as a disease entity." She then began crying. She stated, "Sometimes I feel lucky that I'm ill [with CFS] because I'm really not in the mood to go into work anyway." She also reported disappointment with, and waning interest in, her fiancé. There was a history of other poorly defined medical syndromes during adolescence and an ambivalent relationship with her parents and sister. She offered vivid, rich dream material in the first and subsequent appointments, as described below.

Past Psychiatric History

Miss R. had been treated for 8 months by another psychiatrist with sertraline and Cognitive Behavioral Therapy. The patient denied any improvement in mood or associated symptoms. In addition, she resented the psychiatrist's dismissal of her CFS as "psychosomatic." "He just didn't believe that I had CFS, and he thought it was all in my head." She described those sessions as "like the Socratic method, just arguing back and forth with each other."

Medical History

She had seen several internists who did not confidently endorse the diagnosis of CFS. This frustrated her. She found a specialist in CFS who proposed a theory that she suffered from a "mitochondrial disorder" and prescribed many dietary supplements, which she took regularly. None of these supplements offered any relief.

Family History

Miss R.'s sister was diagnosed with depression by her pediatrician but never received treatment. Miss. R's maternal grandmother committed suicide when Miss. R.'s mother was 12 years old.

171

Substance Use

Miss. R. had tried marijuana while in college a few times but did not continue using it. She reported drinking alcohol in small or moderate amounts at social occasions and denied problems with it.

Developmental History

Childhood and Early Objects: The patient was raised in an upper-middle class suburb of a northeastern metropolitan center by her parents, along with her younger sister. Her father is a professor of mathematics, and her mother a middle school teacher. She describes her mother as "outgoing, overweight but very sexy, bossy, gossipy, likes to sing and to perform, the life of the party. She always talked about sex openly, maybe too openly." She also said, "I know they [her mother and father] have great sex. I can imagine my mother doing it and enjoying it, but I can't even imagine my father taking his clothes off." She describes her father as "brilliant, very logical, cold, controlling, hates emotions, can't understand children, works nonstop." Miss. R.'s parents, particularly her father, dismissed and neglected her needs for physical comfort and emotional dependency: Her father was extremely sensitive to temperature, and the house was kept at only 60° year-round (according to the patient's recollection). The patient and her sister frequently complained of feeling cold but were admonished to "stop whining" and wear a winter coat and scarf in the house. The house was unreasonably dark as her father was very concerned about wasting electricity, and the blinds were kept shut because sunlight would raise the temperature. When she was about 10 years old, a wasp nest was discovered in her bedroom ceiling. She was terrified of being stung and demanded that it be removed immediately, but her father spent 3 to 4 weeks comparing the prices and methods of numerous exterminators before hiring one. Her sister, in contrast to the patient, was doted on as a child because she "always had swollen tonsils and a cough, even though the doctors could never find anything wrong."

Adolescence: Miss R. was a good student and always had friends while growing up. She first had sex at age 16 with her high school boyfriend. She considered herself to have been socially on track in comparison with her peer group. She attended a private liberal arts college, where she had friends and dated casually until she began her next relationship with the young man who was her fiancé at the time of initial presentation. He is a law student at a prestigious university and comes from a wealthy and powerful family.

Current Life Situation: She and her fiancé moved in together once they graduated college and began their respective graduate programs. He is an extravagant young man; he purchases expensive clothing, drives a luxury car, and spends thousands of dollars per month on gambling, expensive video games, and gadgets, etc. He has cheated on law school exams and papers. At the time of initial presentation, she was simultaneously excited by and disapproving of his excesses and "his flexible morality" (her term). She, by contrast, described difficulty purchasing things for herself, such as clothing and new shoes. This came to light when she discussed that she found it extremely difficult to buy a laptop computer, which was a requirement for her graduate studies and teaching. After being accepted into her Ph.D. program, she chose to pursue a research project with a mentor who has a reputation of being the most demanding, harsh, and critical professor in her program. She considers herself to be this professor's "protégée, and favorite student." She was not planning to pursue academics or a career related to mathematics. "I just want to prove that I'm capable of Ph.D. work, but after I get my degree I'll find a different job or stay home and have kids."

COURSE OF TREATMENT

The following two recurrent dreams were offered spontaneously in the first and second appointments.

Dream 1: I'm sitting at the beach with my family, and I stare far out into the ocean, when I see a tidal wave coming for us. I tell my father and my family, and no one believes me. I keep telling them, and nobody listens to me. Then the wave gets much closer, and everyone can see it now. They finally start gathering up all of our things, and it takes so long. It's so frustrating, like when you're trying to fit everything into a bag, but it won't fit. So then, we get all our stuff together, but the beach is really steep. I just couldn't run fast enough. I have to climb up the beach away from the ocean, and when we're just about two-thirds of the way up from the water, the wave gets there and it's about to wash us back out to the ocean, and that's when I wake up. Sometimes we make it as far as the car and on the bridge on the way back from the ocean. I look behind the car and I can still see the waves coming. There's a boy who is climbing a tree and he wants to get away from the waves. Someone pulls down the tree and then lets go, and it sends him flying, like in cartoons. I keep telling my parents that I want to stop and help him, but no one will listen. When we see him, he's in a mangled pool of blood and has bones sticking out of him.

Dream 2: I'm outside and my house is a black rectangle. I don't know where my mother is. My father married our babysitter, who was just a few years older than us. They're upstairs in the bedroom. They had twins, and I'm supposed to be looking after the babies. I'm with the twins outside in the cold, in a giant pit in the snow. A dark figure, like a shadow in an overcoat, comes and kidnaps one of the babies. I tell my father but he doesn't believe me. He says, "Yeah, I'll look around inside here for them, you can look outside." I run after the dark guy, and I chase him over a bridge. I catch up with him and he's holding the baby by the ankles, dangling over the bridge, about to kill him. My father used to hold me like that over the railing by the stairs. My mother was terrified but I used to love it.

In the first few months of therapy, the patient focused on her frustration growing up with her father's aloofness and lack of attention to her feelings or well-being. The patient has often remarked, "My father's attitude was always 'fend for yourselves.'" Miss R. was initially quite ashamed of her feelings of resentment or indignation at her father. She feared that she would be seen as "whining" or "making too much of something." Rather, "I should really just be thankful that my parents provided for me." While growing up, she resented her sister's "playing sick just to get their attention." The babysitter who has appeared in the patient's recurrent dream had a special relationship with her father, in that he tutored her in calculus in exchange for babysitting services while she and her sister were young children.

She continued discussing her father's intellectual style, his impatience for sentiment and emotions, and his inability to express affection. She began to see how she developed a knack for pursuing and discussing things that he'd be interested in. Her drive for academic success in school, which he valued highly, was motivated by her wish for his approval and love. She re-evaluated her feelings about his disdain for expensive and stylish clothing and brand names and his general objection to fun and pleasure. A few months into treatment, anecdotes about her father were less colored by enthusiasm or pleasure and assumed a cruel, sadistic flavor:

Patient: We weren't even allowed to buy any brand names of clothing. He made me feel like I was a horrible, spoiled brat just for wanting an "Alligator-Izod shirt" [i.e., brand-name, stylish clothing]. He never took us seriously when we asked for anything or complained. He hates children. My mother always said that we were the only kids he could tolerate. Sometimes I think she just said that to make us feel better and that maybe he hated all kids, even us.

Her father also hated pets and animals. She and her fiancé "adopted" a bunny during the eighth month of treatment.

Patient: I didn't tell my parents about the bunny. They think pets are stupid. I think about how much my father hates animals, and it makes me sad. He always talked about wanting to poison our neighbor's dog. I don't know why this makes me so sad. I thought I was sad for him, but maybe I'm really sad for me and my sister. He hates when kids need help or cry.
Therapist: It sounds like when you talk about caring for animals, part of you is thinking about caring for children.
Patient: Yeah, I worry sometimes that I'll hate children like my father did. This bunny is like an experiment, sort of a trial run.

She began to re-evaluate her selection of a difficult, critical mentor for her doctoral research and dissertation. Her peers were shocked that would have deliberately chosen this mentor. She explained to her classmates, "She's tough, but I'll learn the most from her." Secretly, she had cherished being this mentor's favorite. As therapy progressed, she began seeing a parallel between her minimizing or overlooking her father's cruelty and coldness, and her deliberate selection of the most unsupportive and difficult professor in the entire department.

She noted when the therapist bought new shoes and shared her interest in his wardrobe and clothing. She also noted that he owned an expensive laptop computer. The therapist invited her to reflect on her thoughts on the fact that he owned these things. She stated, "You're not extravagant like [fiancé] is, but you are not afraid to buy good quality when you own something." She came to an appointment with new clothing, which was not commented on by the therapist. She revealed in the next session that she had hoped the therapist would notice this and had started to wonder if he disapproved of this purchase. The therapist commented, "It sounds like you are proud of yourself for doing something that has been hard for you to do in the past, and you were wondering if I noticed and was proud of you as well." The patient continued to be unsure of the therapist's' "real views" on this. This seemed somewhat implausible, however, since in previous discussions the therapist had revealed his stance that her inability to spend money within her budget on things she legitimately needed was a problem worthy of therapeutic attention. She began speculating on other aspects of the therapist's life, imagining that he was happily married to a beautiful woman who was about to give birth. She initially found the therapist's interest in her dreams and details of her associations during appointments to be puzzling. "This all feels very touchy feely to me," she stated. She also said, "My father would think what you and I are doing here is absolutely crazy. He'd have no idea how this is helping me." She related an additional dream:

Patient: I went to a party at my high school teacher's house. His house looked like your office, though. I was all dirty and wasn't dressed nicely enough for the party. He was a math teacher, but in the dream he was a psychology professor who was doing research with monkeys. He was teaching them how to talk. I had been outside hiking all day in the sun, and I was about to die of thirst. He gave me water and it saved my life.

Miss R. cherished but also felt guilty about her "special status" in the Ph.D. program and her mentor's research group. She imagined that her peers were jealous of her and that they doubted the validity of her CFS. Six months into treatment, the patient began to consider the reality-based possibility of quitting her program. "I know that my father will be so disappointed in me. He thinks the CFS has been totally bogus all along, anyway." She also anticipated disapproval from her fiancé and his mother, who expected her to attain a prestigious degree. Working through this ambivalence, she quit the Ph.D. program in the tenth month of psychotherapy and had an immediate remission of all symptoms of depression and fatigue. She took a job teaching math at a parochial high school and has since been able to work full days without unusual fatigue or problems. She commented, "I wondered whether you really believed in CFS at the beginning. If you had said you believed me, I wouldn't have respected you. It's like I was ready to get into a fight with you about it." She also noted, "I originally assumed that you thought I should finish my Ph.D. It was really eye-opening that, if anything, you seemed to approve of me quitting."

She began talking more about her mother. She had long been annoyed by her mother's boisterous and provocative style ("always the center of attention"), but she started to appreciate her mother as being affectionate and warm. She ultimately considered her mother to be "happier and more balanced" than her father. She was no longer angry at her sister but began worrying about her. She attempted to obtain a referral for her sister to see a psychotherapist for a consultation, but the sister refused. She experienced deep sadness about the fact she would "never feel very close" to her father, and she feared her sister "might never lead a normal, happy life." Her difficulties with her fiancé increased, however. She grew annoyed by his extravagance. She learned that he was having an affair with another woman and she ended the engagement. She expressed romantic interest in a male friend from college. They began dating. She discussed a fantasy of getting pregnant accidentally and quickly getting married.

Therapy was conducted twice weekly for 16 months. Therapy was concluded when the psychiatrist moved to another city, and referral was made for continued therapy with the psychiatrist's colleague, which the patient pursued.

CASE DISCUSSION AND FORMULATION

Not all patients discuss their dreams, but when they do it can be a special opportunity to learn about unconscious wishes and affects. This patient's dreams serve as an example of this, and a brief discussion of her dreams will shed light on many other aspects of her presentation. In both dreams, children are in serious danger. She attempts to elicit the attention of her father or her parents, but she is not taken seriously. Her house is caricatured as a dark rectangle, and she is, metaphorically, "left out in the cold." The babysitter, who in fact had a special relationship with the patient's father, is upstairs in the bedroom, suggesting a sexual relationship. The patient is aware of having felt jealous of this babysitter. The babysitter, therefore, functions in the dream as a masked representation of her mother; the patient is ignored by her father while he is upstairs in the bedroom with an older woman who has functioned as her caretaker. Of course, the patient is unaware of this conflict on a conscious level, and simply recalls having a puzzling, recurrent dream. In addition, the baby being dangled over a bridge is very reminiscent of the game her father played with her as a child over their stairwell. This is a reflection of her repressed awareness about her father that this type of "horseplay" is actually an expression of sadistic cruelty.

There are two painful aspects of the patient's longing for her father's love: 1) It pins her in conflict against her mother, whom she also loves. 2) Her love for him feels to her as though it is unrequited because he has been cold and not at all attuned to her emotional happiness or physical well-being. She defends herself against these painful affects in a number of ways. She represses her rivalry with her mother. This rivalry shows up in a peculiar dream she herself does not understand—her mother is not present in the dream, but is instead masked, symbolically, by the babysitter. This substitution prevents her from becoming aware of her hostile feelings toward her mother which are agitated by envy over their sexual intimacy. She also represses the sexual dimension of her longing for her father, which is evident in her limited capacity to see him as a sexual man, as opposed to her ability to vividly imagine her mother's sexuality. She shows some impaired judgment regarding her ability to choose a suitable mentor in her graduate studies and research. She has deliberately chosen the most harsh and critical mentor, whom others in her program have understandably decided to avoid. She shows the defenses of *rationalization* (i.e., explains her choice of this mentor as though there are plausible, logical reasons for choosing a critical and unsupportive boss) and *reaction formation* (i.e., reframes her reactions from dread or horror into excitement and enthusiasm as a means of avoiding unpleasant effects). This may represent an unconscious desire to be punished (referred to as *masochism*)—there is something gratifying to her about having a harsh mentor who is cruel to her, similar to her "enjoyment" of her father dangling her as a little girl by her feet over a stairwell.

Her view of her fiancé appears to be organized around his extravagance and "flexible morality." She enjoys his tendency to pamper himself, but at the same time recognizes that he is dishonest and spoiled. This might be an attempt to choose an object that is different from her father, but this particular young man's excesses are unreasonable and ultimately cause the relationship to fail. Early psychoanalytic authors described a phenomenon when young men who have a very intense relationship with their mothers are unable to feel sexual attraction to women who are from their same socio-economic background. They attempt to date and marry "suitable women" but are much more attracted to "women of ill repute." This is referred to as "whore-Madonna splitting." This is also observed in young women, who are attracted to "bad boys." As another patient succinctly explained this, "The kinds of guys that are fun to 'fool around' with [i.e., engage in sexual relations with] are not the same guys I can bring home to Mommy and Daddy." The patient's choice of a man who is an exaggerated caricature of the *opposite* of her father's personality and beliefs may well represent a type of whore-Madonna splitting.

From the point of view of wishes, defenses, and conflicts, the following is observed: The patient's "chronic fatigue syndrome" relates to her conflict over quitting the Ph.D. program. On the one hand, she wants to complete the program and fulfill what she imagines to be her father's expectations that she will become a successful mathematician. On the other hand, she has a hostile mentor who makes her feel inadequate when she shows up to work. (Furthermore, she is not even interested in a career in mathematics!) Therefore by developing "chronic fatigue syndrome" which prevents her from attending classes and her research responsibilities, the patient has found a way simultaneously both to quit her program (a forbidden wish) and to try heroically to attend classes despite feeling ill (the denial of this wish). A behavior which partially expresses a forbidden wish and simultaneously expresses the defense against that wish is called a *compromise formation*. The patient's psychosomatic illness is a *compromise formation* between her desire to end the program, and her shame and guilt about not living up to what she imagines (perhaps correctly) is required to gain her father's respect or admiration.

Similarities between the patient's father and the patient's research mentor (both are harsh, critical, unsupportive) suggests another defensive phenomenon which was described originally by Freud: the *repetition compulsion*. Patients who utilize this mechanism of defense are unconsciously attracted to the same situations—they are *compelled* to *repeat* earlier traumas. The explanation offered by psychoanalytic thinking for this phenomenon is a wish to master conflicts and challenges—to "get it right this time." There is likely an unconscious fantasy that *this time* she will win over her father and finally receive the love and affection she needs to believe is present for her. The mentor thus serves as a symbolic representation of her father. It is essentially the same struggle. She attempts to conform to what she imagines her father or mentor will be pleased with.

Lester Luborsky, a prominent writer and teacher of psychoanalytic psychotherapy, has observed that many patients find themselves entangled in the same interpersonal conflict repeatedly throughout life and that many of a patient's problems can be well explained by identifying how they are re-enacting the same drama which they experienced in early relationships with parents, siblings, or other important figures in their lives. This is an application of Freud's idea of the *repetition compulsion* to an object relations model. Luborsky's apt term for this concept is the "Core Conflictual Relationship Theme" (CCRT). In the present case, there is a relationship theme which is organized around the patient struggling with people over the question of her physical needs being taken seriously and whether they can tolerate her emotional dependency and need for support or reassurance. Her father ignored the presence of a wasp nest in her room, showed no concern for her normal adolescent female desire to wear stylish clothing, kept the house at an uncomfortably low temperature, etc. Her previous psychiatrist doubted the legitimacy of her Chronic Fatigue Syndrome diagnosis and she experienced him as openly accusing her of "making it all up." She imagined that her father similarly felt this diagnosis was "bogus." She tested the current therapist in the very first session to see whether he, too, would doubt her beliefs. She later acknowledged that she would not have believed the therapist had he professed to credulously accept the veracity of her Chronic Fatigue Diagnosis. Therefore, from the point of view of interpersonal relationships, the same pattern (a struggle over being taken seriously and being nurtured and cared for physically) is present with her father since childhood, with her research mentor, her fiancé, and in the transference toward her psychotherapist. That is, this drama is present in three spheres: *the past* (father), *the present* (mentor and fiancé), and the *transference* (both the present and previous psychotherapist). When the same interpersonal struggle is repeatedly present in a patient who shows relatively high social and occupational functioning, many psychotherapists would identify this as a very fruitful focus for potential therapeutic change.

From a self psychology perspective, we would focus on how the patient's feelings, thoughts, and behavior serve to help maintain and promote a positive sense of her self-worth, identity, abilities, stability, and safety over time. The patient is clearly concerned that others will think she is exaggerating her illnesses, shirking her responsibilities, complaining, or whining. These all represent the numerous negative self-representations which are operating in her at any given time. Much of her anxiety and behavior can be explained by a fear of being "unmasked" as a needy, weak, whining nuisance, which appears to be her sense of what her father feels about her. Intelligence, hard work, sound logic, and clear thinking are attributes which the patient has attributed to herself over time. These appear to have been the attributes for which she has successfully obtained positive feedback from both parents, as well as from teachers, who also occasionally appear in her dreams. Academic success has served as an external marker for these attributes. Obtaining a graduate degree even though she has no plans to make professional use of it appears to be motivated by a need to maintain her view of herself as a productive, competent, and highly intelligent woman.

Outline and Worksheet for Bio-Psycho-Social Psychotherapy Case Formulation

Patient: <u>Miss R.</u>   *Date:* <u>March, 2003–June, 2004.</u>
*Therapist:*_____

1. BIOLOGICAL FACTORS

 a. Family psychiatric history and genetic vulnerability to psychiatric conditions:
  Maternal grandmother suffered depression and committed suicide. Sister diagnosed with depression.

 b. Birth and developmental history, head injuries, other neurological problems, past and current medical conditions, and their impact on psychiatric illness and symptoms:
  "Chronic fatigue syndrome" at time of initial presentation, but otherwise unremarkable.

 c. Current medications and their impact on psychiatric illness and symptoms:
  None at time of presentation. Prior antidepressants (paroxetine, sertraline) were not helpful.

 d. Substance use/misuse and its impact on psychiatric illness and symptoms:
  Unremarkable.

2. SOCIAL FACTORS

 a. Financial situation (monthly income, source of income, monthly expenses):
  Very low monthly expenses, lives on graduate student stipend, has savings available in case of emergency, has access to some financial support from fiancé and parents if need be as well.

b. Employment (job stability, relationship with boss/coworkers, work-related stress or other problems):

Research mentor in graduate program is critical, unsupportive, and harsh. Afraid of being thrown out of program at time of initial presentation because of poor attendance. Left program during treatment and obtained full-time position teaching in private high school.

c. Supportive relationships (or lack thereof/social isolation) (Are friends, family, or neighbors available to help patient with errands, child care, etc?):

Numerous friends, fiancé. Friends not aware of how badly patient is feeling.

d. Recent disruption of relationships (break-ups, divorce, people who have moved out of town, and how is patient coping):

Discovered fiancé was cheating on her and patient ended the relationship during treatment.

e. Other recent losses/grief:

None.

f. Legal problems:

None.

g. Crises in lives of important people in patient's life: (health, financial, or legal problems in relatives/partner/friends):

None.

h. Access to medical and psychiatric care, affordability of proposed treatment:

Student health insurance pays for treatment at university. After leaving university, was able to afford co-pays with new insurance. Fortunately, generous policy covered twice weekly visits.

3. PSYCHOLOGICAL FACTORS

a. Drives and ego functions (see worksheet)

b. Object relations (see worksheet)

c. Self psychology (see worksheet)

a. Drives and Ego Functions

Symptoms, negative feelings, reported difficulties, other problems	Defenses and Coping Mechanisms	Underlying or disavowed wishes, drives, or beliefs against which the defenses are directed	Superego admonitions against disavowed wishes	How successful are these defenses or coping mechanisms? How aware is patient of underlying wishes? Is reality testing preserved? How are these defenses helpful or adaptive? What problems do they cause?
Recurrent dream about babysitter, as above. Inability to imagine father's sexuality. Frustration and annoyance at mother. Choosing a fiancé exactly unlike her father.	*Repression (Unconscious wishes and feelings are buried into unconsciousness.)*	*Desire for love and intimacy with father, envy of mother's sexual intimacy with him.*	*Taboo against incestuous fantasies; sting of rejection by father; guilt about hostility toward mother, whom she loves; threat of losing relationship with mother.*	*Patient is able to avoid acknowledgment of unconscious wishes, which (though postulated by psychoanalytic thinkers to be ubiquitous) would be distressing for anyone to acknowledge. Also avoids feelings of rejection by father. Maladaptive, as her inability to understand how severely she longs for father leads her to make poorly informed decisions. Also, distances self from mother unnecessarily.*
Choosing the most difficult and harsh research supervisor (graduate mentor) in her entire department.	*Rationalization ("She's tough, but I'll learn a lot from her." "No pain, no gain.")* *Repetition compulsion: trying to master the struggle with her father.* *Masochism: deriving pleasure from being beaten, punished.*	*It would be rebellious or disrespectful to identify her mentor (or father) as inappropriately harsh, critical, cold, etc.*		*Allows her to avoid considering how problematic father's way of relating to her really is. Enables her to continue fantasy that she will win over her father and receive love, affection from him. Maladaptive in*

(continues)

185

a. Drives and Ego Functions (continued)

			that she makes poor decisions and chooses an unnecessarily difficult supervisor.
Inability to attend work, fatigue, "chronic fatigue syndrome."	*Rationalization, compromise formation.*	*Father's expectations will not be met. Patient would fail to fulfill her own ideals of hard work and academic success. She will feel like a quitter.*	*Desire to quit graduate program.* / *This defense prevents patient from experiencing pain of letting her father down and failing to meet her own low expectations. They are maladaptive in that patient's inability to acknowledge her desire to stop her graduate studies prevents her from making a good decisions and keeps her perpetually locked in a situation where she "tries" to complete her studies, but "simply can't make it to class" because of her fatigue symptoms.*
Difficulty spending money on herself, buying nice clothing, etc.	*Reaction Formation— (An unconscious impulse is kept out of awareness by conversion into the exact opposite of the true, underlying wish.)*	*Belief that it is an expression of strength and virtue to withstand temptation, and (conversely) a manifestation of gluttony and immorality to consume more than absolutely necessary.*	*Greed and wish to for oral gratification; desire to consume things.* / *Patient avoids acknowledging greed and related wishes which she finds unacceptable about herself. This is maladaptive in that her disavowal of normal human desires is so severe that she is unable to purchase even necessary things without guilt and distress. In addition, dressing well and cultivating a nice appearance can be important skills in life.*

(continues)

b. Object Relations (Impact of Relationships on Internal Mental Life)

Objects (parents or caregiver, siblings, spouse, peers, boss, mentors, or other important persons in the patient's life)	Characterize this relationship over time. Describe the success or lack thereof of early and sustained *attachment* to this object, *unmet needs, ungratified wishes, conflicts,* and struggles.	Does this relationship fall into a typical pattern or theme which is comparable with the other relationships listed?	Does the patient's <u>transference</u> to the psychotherapist resemble this relationship? How does the therapist respond (*counter-transference or enactments*) to the patient's transference?
Father	Patient has had an ongoing struggle with attaining affection and other manifestations of love from her father. She has experienced him as uninterested in her physical well-being and safety, and annoyed at her for asking for these needs to be met. She has gone out of her way to pursue activities and cultivate talents which will impress him. She is inhibited from making decisions that he would disapprove of (e.g., making expensive purchases, leaving graduate school).	*This is the prototypical relationship which has become the reference point for many other relationships in her life.*	*Compared and contrasted therapist with father openly. Attributed to therapist same disapproving and critical attitude toward her desire for new clothing then revised this. Tested therapist at beginning of treatment to see if he would take seriously her physical well-being.*
Fiancé	He is a person who has been able to gratify his greed longings for pleasure with seemingly no inhibitions. He also shows major problems with honesty and reliability as a partner. She is stimulated by his ability indulge his wishes and desires with no remorse or guilt,	He appears to represent the exact opposite of her father. She has chosen a man who acts out her forbidden wishes. Spending resembles mother.	*Patient also projects unfulfilled wishes and fantasies onto therapist, becoming fascinated by his spending habits. After leaving fiancé due to*

(continues)

187

b. Object Relations (Impact of Relationships on Internal Mental Life) (continued)

	but she disapproves of his lack of an internalized sense of morality or ethics.	*infidelity, she fantasized that therapist is a devoted family man.*
Graduate advisor/ research mentor	The patient selected this mentor out of a group of numerous faculty members. All of the classmates have avoided this mentor because she is so critical and hostile. Patient took pride in being this professor's "protégée." However, patient felt criticized, constantly rejected, and undervalued by this mentor over time. Found it very difficult to acknowledge how negative and unsupportive this relationship was. Patient stopped attending work due to "chronic fatigue," testing this mentor to see if she'd believe and support her, or dismiss her.	Also a mathematician. Same essential struggle as that with father. Tries to win over a harsh and critical person. Tests object's concern for her well-being.	*Patient tested therapist at the outset of treatment in a very similar manner. Wondered if he "believes in CFS" (i.e., if he believes in her).*
Mother	Patient initially resented mother's emotional demonstratives and dramatics. Resented mother's "seeking attention all the time." Saw mother as a spendthrift who had excessive and extravagant tastes.	Has applied father's standards to her view of mother—sees her as foolish and "over-emotional."	*Was also initially uncomfortable with the therapist's interest in her dreams and feelings. She found it difficult to accept his position that she should be more flexible with money and buying things. (i.e., she was uncomfortable with the maternal and empathic position of the therapist.)*

c. Self Psychology

Self-representations: (Included are common examples of important self-representations. Other terms may be better for a specific patient.)	Selfobjects (Identify important people, activities, possessions, etc., that influence the patient's self-representations.)	Selfobject transferences (i.e., how does this selfobject influence the patient's self-representations, e.g., mirroring, idealizing, twin/alter-ego transferences?)	Defensive and compensatory mechanisms (i.e., what does the patient do in response to these self-representations and the emotional impact of these self-objects—is this response adaptive, maladaptive?)
Patient sees herself as whining, undisciplined, unproductive. Feels physically vulnerable but unworthy of being cared for. Feels dependent and despicable for not being more independent.	*Father*	*Father has made her feel guilty for asking to have physical needs met. E.g., reluctance to remove wasp nest from room; insistence on keeping house at cold temperature are not isolated incidents, but are emblematic of a long standing pattern whereby it was conveyed to patient that she has no right to expect to be cared for. Father hates animals, that are symbolic of dependent children. Mirroring, and Identification.*	*Patient has dealt with these feelings about herself by internalizing her father's values and has attempted to live up to them by adopting a stoic and disciplined life and by taking on significant challenges. This has helped her attain a degree of academic success but stifles her freedom to live a different, more satisfying life.*
Patient sees herself as not living up to her intellectual and productive potential.	*Father Mentor*	*Mentor is very critical and harsh. Father has exacting standards and is very disapproving of people who are "too emotional," "stupid," or "illogical." Mirroring, and identification.*	*Patient adopts these standards and applies them toward herself. Similar as above, motivates her for academic and intellectual accomplishments, but limits her choices and freedom.*

(continues)

189

c. Self Psychology (continued)

Sees self as gluttonous, greedy, extravagant, and spoiled.	Fiancé	Fiancé acts out her unconscious fantasies. She is excited by but ashamed of his behavior. This represents an <u>alter-ego transference</u>.
	Father	Father has expressed disapproval of her desire for brand name clothing, etc.	Chose a boyfriend who allowed her to vicariously act out these unconscious wishes. At the same time, she adopted her father's values. She avoids buying nice things, disavows her own desires and greed.
Sees self as intelligent, productive.	Academic success throughout her career. Teachers from earlier in life, current research mentor.	Patient has been an outstanding student and worked very hard to get into a prestigious Ph.D. program of which she is very proud. Teachers have always given her very positive feedback. (One teacher appeared in a recent dream.) Current mentor, the most difficult in the department, considers patient to be "her protégé." <u>Mirroring, identification.</u>	When she realizes that she does not want to become a mathematician after all, she still attempts to stay in the program so as not to lose her special "protégé" status. Even after she leaves the program, she takes a job as a math teacher, thus deepening her identification with teachers who have given her positive feedback since childhood.
Sees self as a potentially loving and nurturing wife and mother, though she is somewhat unsure about this.	Mother Pet rabbit Sister Therapist	Through psychotherapy, better able to appreciate her mother's warmth and affection. She "adopts" a rabbit as a "trial run" for taking care of children. She experiences therapist as interested in and encouraging of her cultivation of these qualities.	She had initially feared that she lacked capacity to function as a mother. She distanced herself from her mother and identified with father's peculiar and stoic traits. With therapy, began to explore her maternal side, became concerned about her younger sister.

190

4. PROPOSED TREATMENT:

a. Medications (category, agent, dose, goals for symptom improvement, and method/plan for monitoring symptoms):

Patient appears to manifest a genetic predisposition to depression. She was started on venlafaxine extended release and titrated to 225mg/day.

b. Social interventions (connection with social service agencies, notification of Child Protective Services, or Adult Protective Services, etc.):

Therapist wrote letter on her behalf stating that she suffered from depression which she handed in to her graduate program administrators to document reasons for absences.

c. Psychotherapy

i. Modality of therapy:

Psychodynamic psychotherapy with aim of helping patient become more aware of the numerous forces at work inside of her which are preventing her from considering a full range of options open to her.

ii. Length of treatment (open-ended vs. time-limited, number of sessions anticipated):

Therapist anticipates graduating from his training program in 16 months. Patient's problems are numerous enough and impact multiple areas of functioning to justify an open-ended course of treatment. Sixteen months was felt to be sufficient time for substantial progress even though all issues might not be fully addressed.

iii. Issues of focus (related to above issues in the formulation):

1. *Symptoms of Major Depressive Episode.*
2. *Ambivalence over completing Ph.D. program.*
3. *Problematic relationship with research mentor.*
4. *Problematic relationship with father.*

5. *Harsh views of herself*
6. *Deliberately decided to avoid focusing on chronic fatigue syndrome, which appeared to be a potential pitfall for confirming patient's sense that no one believes her or takes her seriously and would likely sabotage this therapy just as it did with previous therapist.*

iv. Current or anticipated transferences and countertransferences
   1. *That patient will presume that therapist does not believe her or take seriously her symptoms of chronic fatigue syndrome.*
   2. *That patient will presume that therapist expects her to complete her graduate program and will be disappointed if she does not.*
   3. *That therapist will be uncomfortable when patient attributes harshness and criticism to him.*

d. Consultations with other professionals (M.D. for medication evaluation, psychologist for neuropsychological testing, primary care physician or medical/surgical specialist for evaluation/treatment):
None indicated.

FINAL COMMENTS

Multiple perspectives were utilized over the course of this psychotherapy treatment. Each perspective contributed to understanding the patient's problems and planning her psychotherapy treatment in different ways. In the initial formulation and treatment planning, drives the ego's mechanisms of defenses (especially Oedipal conflict) were evident in the presenting clinical phenomenology. Over the course of her treatment, helping the patient understand repetitive relationship patterns (object relations) proved to be the most useful single intervention for much of the therapeutic work. Toward the end of the therapy, the patient began to understand how she had internalized some of her father's values and beliefs, and re-examined her view of herself. Specifically, she re-evaluated her self-representations as greedy and spoiled and began to think of herself as a loving and nurturing woman and future mother. This phase of treatment can be best described by a self-psychological perspective.

Formulating a case from multiple points of view can be a powerful exercise because it forces the therapist to think of multiple, possible interventions for the same psychological problems. After numerous possibilities are considered, the psychotherapist has a wider range of options in his or her therapeutic armamentarium.

RECOMMENDED READINGS

Baker HS, and Baker MN. Heinz Kohut's Self Psychology: An Overview. *American Journal of Psychiatry.* January, 1987: 144(1):1–9.

Freud S. On the universal tendency to debasement in the sphere of love. In Strachey J, ed-trans. *The Standard Edition of the Complete Psychological Works of Sigmund Freud.* Vol 11. London: Hogarth Press, 1961: 179–190. [on the Whore-Madonna complex]

Freud S. Beyond the pleasure principle. In Strachey, J, ed-trans. *The Standard Edition of the Complete Psychological Works of Sigmund Freud* Vol 18. London: Hogarth Press, 1961: 7–64. [On the repetition compulsion]

Luborsky L. *Understanding Transference: The Core Conflictual Relationship Theme Method.* American Psychological Association, 1997.

Pine F. *Drive, Ego, Object, and Self: A Synthesis for Clinical Work.* New York: Basic Books, 1990.

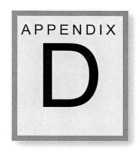

APPENDIX

D

Comparison of Psychodynamic and Cognitive Models

	Psychodynamic	Cognitive
Healthy mental function	Drive, ego, object relations Coherent structures managing drive derivatives Self Cohesive self, healthy narcissism	Accurate perception of meaning of events Conscious choice of responses
Proximate sources of pathology	Drive Id impulses overwhelm ego Ego Conflicts between defenses; conflicts between drives and defenses Object relations Maladaptive perceptions of objects Primitive splitting Self Breakdown products of inadequately cohesive self	Cognitive distortions (e.g., black-and-white thinking, taking matters too personally, pessimistic predictions) Conditional assumptions and compensatory strategies based on negative core beliefs
Root sources of pathology	Drive Repressed drive impulses Ego Inadequate defense mechanisms Object relations Distorted or imbalanced object world Self Imbalance of grandiose and idealizing poles of self	Negative core beliefs, resulting from temperament and environment

Aims of therapy	<u>Drive, ego</u> Balance of ego defenses against drive urges and superego demands Relief of neurotic symptoms <u>Object relations</u> Adaptive perceptions of, and interactions with, others Minimization of splitting Affective stability <u>Self</u> Restoration of balance between grandiose and idealized poles of self Empathy, creativity, humor, wisdom, acceptance of mortality	Relief of affective symptoms Control of maladaptive behavior Substitution of conscious choices for automatic responses Correction of negative core beliefs
Foci of therapeutic investigation	Historical roots of current pathology Unconscious determinants of affect and symptoms Meanings of environmental events	Automatic thoughts Meanings of environmental events
Major therapeutic modalities	Free association Confrontation and clarification Interpretation	Confrontation and clarification Provocative inquiry Behavioral assignments
Role of transference	Primary focus of investigation and interpretation	Examined as example of automatic thoughts when reactions impede therapy

Index

Page numbers followed by f indicate figures; t, tables.

Neurosis
    definition, 153
    Horney's view of, 68–70
    transference, 120
Normal autism, 77–78

O

Object relations
    comparison with other perspectives,
        133t–135t
    narcissism and, 22–24
    and psychodynamic formulation,
        169, 187–188
    theory of, 73–87, 106–114
        comparison of major theories, 86t
        D.W. Winnicott, true and false
            selves, 81–83
        Margaret Mahler, 77–79, 108–109
        Melanie Klein, 75–77, 107–108
        Otto Kernberg, 83–84, 109–111
        principles common to, 75t
        refinement of theories, 85
        W.R.D. Fairbairn, 79–81, 109
    therapeutic implications, 132,
        136–145
Object-seeking, studied by W.R.D.
    Fairbairn, 79–81
Oedipal conflicts, 123
Oedipal crisis, 14–16
    definition, 153
Opposites
    interplay of, 43–45
    principle of, 41
Optimal frustration, 94
    definition, 153
Oral character types, 104
Oral personalities, 13–14
Oral phase, 13

P

Pampering, effects of, 32
Paranoia, 101–102
Paranoid position, 76
    definition, 153
Parapraxes, 17, 20–22
    definition, 153
Part objects, 23
Perfection, striving for, 30
Persona, 43
Personality types, 13–14
Personal unconscious, 39
Phallic personalities, 14
Phallic phase, 13
Practicing, 78

Preconscious system, 9t
    definition, 153
Primary process, 12
    definition, 153
Psychic determinism, 7–8
    definition, 153
Psychoanalysis
    fundamental hypotheses, 7–8
    historical origins, 5–7
    interpersonal, 65–71
    rules of, 123–124
Psychodynamic formulation
    biology and social environment,
        161–193
    comprehensive, 159–193
    jargon and technical language,
        160–161
Psychodynamic models, comparison
    with cognitive model, 196–197
Psychodynamic theory, contributors
    to, 156–158
Psychological development, 11–13
Psychopathology
    studied by Adler, 34–36
    theory, affect, and, 97–98
Psychosocial development, Erikson's
    stages of, 59t

R

Rapprochement, 78, 137
Regression, 104, 141–142, 148
Repression, shadow and, 43–44
Resistance analysis, 147
Rules of psychoanalysis, 123–124

S

Satisfaction, Sullivan's theory
    regarding, 67
Secondary process, 12
    definition, 153
Secondary revision, definition, 154
Security, Sullivan's theory regarding,
    67
Self
    bipolar, 91–93
    in Horney's view of neurosis, 69–70
    role in Jung's theory, 44–45
    and selfobjects, 90–91
    true and false, 81–83
Selfobject
    deficits, 113–114
    definition, 154
    mirroring, 91, 113
    self and, 90–91